FASTING FOR A HEALTHY LIFESTYLE & EXTREME WEIGHT LOSS 2 IN 1 BOOK: ONE MEAL A DAY INTERMITTENT FASTING + WATER FASTING

A BEGINNER'S GUIDE FOR A FASTING FOCUSED LIFESTYLE TO GET HEALTHY AND LOSE WEIGHT EFFORTLESSLY

KATE MCCARTHY

DOWNLOAD YOUR FREE CHEAT SHEET

(Don't start fasting before you've consulted this cheat sheet...)

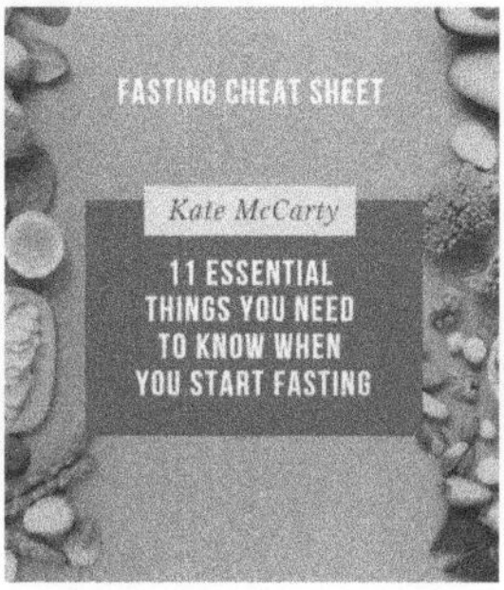

This cheat sheet includes:

- 11 things to know and to do while you are fasting.
- Why you need to know those things to start successfully.
- These things will make the process easier and more enjoyable.

The last thing I want is that the fasting process will be uncomfortable.

To receive your fasting cheat sheet, scan this QR code:

CONTENTS

ONE MEAL A DAY INTERMITTENT FASTING

WATER FASTING

ONE MEAL A DAY INTERMITTENT FASTING

HOW TO LOSE WEIGHT EFFORTLESSLY, IMPROVE YOUR HEALTH, INCREASE MENTAL CLARITY, ACTIVATE AUTOPHAGY, AND HAVE MORE ENERGY

INTRODUCTION: THE INTERMITTENT FASTING TREND

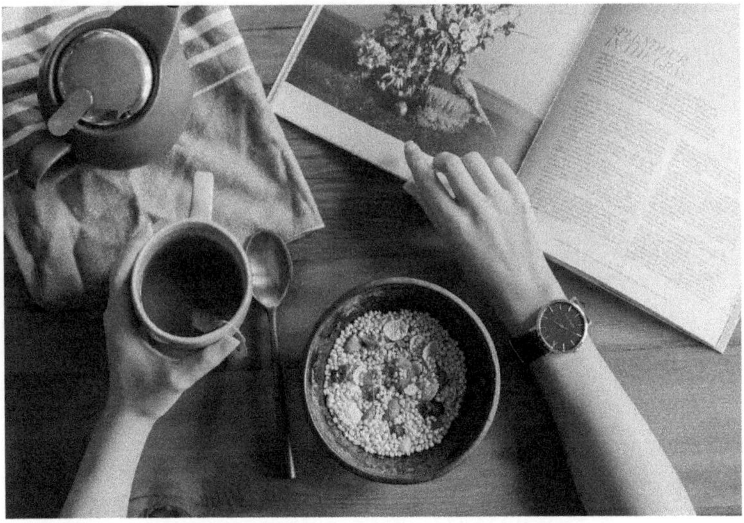

Fig. 1: IF. Pixabay, by The 5th, 2016, https://pixabay.com/photos/breakfast-healthy-food-diet-fruit-1663295/ Copyright 2016 by The 5th/Pixabay.

> *"Fasting is the first principle of medicine; fast and see the strength of the spirit reveal itself."*
>
> — RUMI

Are you tired of the endless diets you have been following that don't seem to be doing anything to improve your health? Or are you interested in making a significant change in your diet, and you're looking for the best option out there?

No matter what your reasons are for picking up this book, you're about to learn a lot of interesting information that can change your life for the better. You may have already heard about the intermittent fasting trend. After all, people all over the world are following intermittent fasting or "IF" and raving about how great their journeys are since they followed this eating pattern. The fact is, intermittent fasting isn't a diet—it's more of an eating pattern or lifestyle that comes with its own rules and guidelines.

If you're interested in learning about IF, specifically about the One Meal A Day (OMAD) method, then you have just chosen the best book for your health journey. Intermittent fasting is a powerful eating pattern that provides so many health benefits when followed correctly. Physiologically speaking, when you restrict your caloric intake by fasting intermittently, this can help increase your lifespan while improving your resistance to several metabolic factors that cause stress to the body (Hine, et. al., 2014). Evidence of this has been seen in studies conducted on animals, although more research is needed on humans to solidify this fact. However, those who support intermittent fasting believe that it can cause a special kind of immune response that repairs the cells of the body while stimulating several positive metabolic changes too.

Another essential benefit of intermittent fasting is weight-loss. This also happens to be one of the most common reasons why people decide to follow IF. Although other methods of fasting aren't associated with sustainable weight loss results, intermittent fasting works differently. As you follow this eating pattern, it gives your body an automatic caloric deficit, thus, promoting the burning of fat in your body. It also boosts your metabolism in the process and prevents you from getting cravings during your fasting windows. According to research, it promotes fat loss instead of water weight or muscle mass compared to dietary detoxes, cleanses, or extremely low-calorie diets. In fact, one review has shown that IF can help you lose up to 7% of your waist circumference in less than two months (Barnosky, et. al., 2014). This means that fat loss occurs in the belly, which is very beneficial as belly fat can cause harm to your organs.

These are just some of the benefits you can look forward to when you start intermittent fasting. There are many more that we will be discussing later. One thing I can tell you right now is that intermittent fasting isn't a strict eating pattern that will make you feel deprived. There are different methods for following IF and you can choose the best way to suit your lifestyle. Because of this flexibility, the technique that makes the most sense to you can be your new method for eating throughout the day.

Typically, intermittent fasting involves alternate periods of eating (feeding windows) with periods of fasting (fasting windows). While fasting, you wouldn't consume any solids, but you can have non-caloric beverages like water, tea, and coffee. Sometimes, you can even have a bowl of broth if you're feeling really hungry. When it comes to IF, you don't focus on restricting or eliminating certain foods from your diet. Instead, you would focus more on your eating schedule. But before we go any further, let me share my story and how intermittent fasting has changed my life. Hopefully, this can inspire you to keep reading so that you can learn everything about this eating pattern and how it can change your life for the better too.

When I was in my early 20s, I started suffering from insulin resistance. Since I was so young, this came as a shock to me. This condition increased my risk of developing diabetes, and it also affected my weight. Although I wasn't particularly health-conscious before getting diagnosed with insulin resistance, I was pretty confident about my diet and health habits. Despite this, I had to start taking medications to prevent my condition from getting worse. However, regardless of the medicinal and diet interventions I had, my insulin sensitivity didn't improve enough for me to get my previous life back. Knowing this was very hard for me. At such a young age, I already had a condition that I felt would ruin the rest of my life.

Instead of giving up, I decided to make healthier life choices. Since medications weren't helping me in the big way that I thought they would, I started researching holistic and alternative practices when I turned 30. By then, I was already suffering for years, both physically and psychologically. I knew that I had to do something to make things better so that I wouldn't experience depression. Through my research, I had come across intermittent fasting. At the time, it was one of the emerging trends in the diet world, and from the first time I had read about it, I was hooked.

In particular, I was very interested in the One Meal A Day approach, otherwise known as OMAD. As a person who leads a hectic and unpredictable lifestyle, the OMAD method of intermittent fasting seemed very interesting to me. I felt like it would fit my routine perfectly. Of course, the OMAD method was very different from my then-current eating habits. Through my research, I knew that forcing myself to follow this method right away would cause more problems for me, healthwise.

Since I had never tried fasting before, I took things slowly. I learned all the methods of IF and how to do them. Then I chose the most basic method and started incorporating it into my routine. It was definitely a change for me, and I did experience all of the things I had read about. To make things easier, I focused on choosing the right foods to eat during my feeding windows to ensure that I was getting all the nutrients my body needed to stay healthy. I also started practicing meditation and mindfulness, which made the journey easier too. I had the determination to commit to this eating pattern and after some time, I saw concrete results. Amazingly, I was able to lose a total of 50 pounds from the weight I gained because of my insulin resistance!

Apart from this, my doctors also told me that my condition had improved so much since I started IF that they gave me the go-signal to stop taking medications! This piece of news made me over-the-moon happy. It also inspired me to write this book and another one about Water Fasting, another highly effective method that has helped me achieve my health and diet goals. Whether you are experiencing the same situation I experienced, or you just want to make positive changes in your life, I hope this book can help you out. Here, I summed up everything I learned when I researched about intermittent fasting and the OMAD method.

As someone who has suffered through a medical condition that changed my life drastically, I wrote this book with compassion and love. Throughout my journey, I received no less from my friends and family, so now, I want to pay it forward by helping others get through their struggles. No matter what your struggles are right now, I hope that this book will help transform your life for the better. By learning about IF here, I hope that you can start following this amazing eating pattern so that you can experience the health improvements that are hidden in such simple practices.

1

YOUR BODY ON INTERMITTENT FASTING

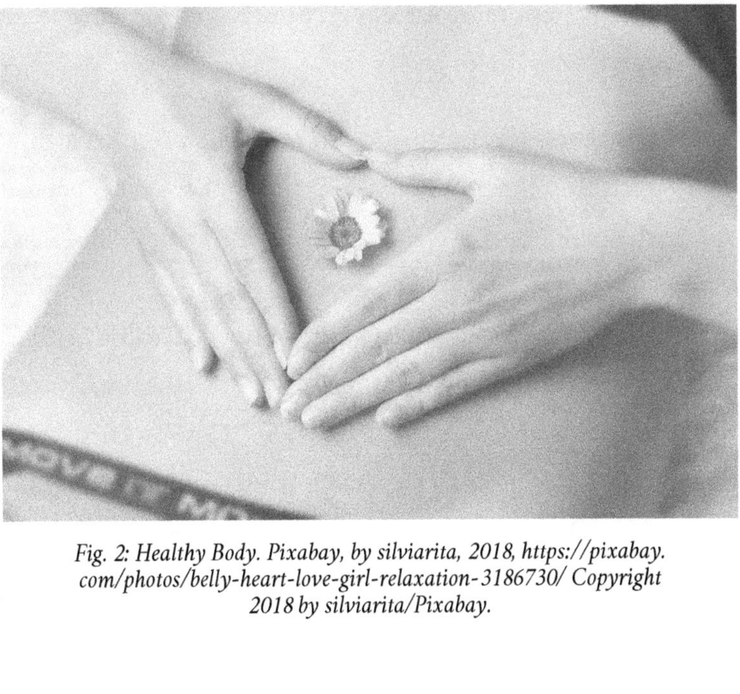

Fig. 2: Healthy Body. Pixabay, by silviarita, 2018, https://pixabay.com/photos/belly-heart-love-girl-relaxation-3186730/ Copyright 2018 by silviarita/Pixabay.

Intermittent fasting is a unique eating pattern that can potentially benefit your health in different ways. In fact, there are so many research studies conducted on IF and its effects, and most of these show promising results. Usually, the animal subjects and even the human participants of these studies have experienced weight loss and an improvement in their cholesterol levels. Researchers found that it can even be used as part of the treatment for certain conditions. While most of these studies have been conducted on rats, almost all studies on humans have also shown that IF is both effective and safe. More importantly, choosing the right method of IF can make this eating pattern more effective, realistic, and sustainable for you to reach your health goals.

Although fasting has already been a concept since the dawn of time, recently, IF has become one of the more popular approaches for losing weight. Different forms of fasting have existed for ages, especially as a tool for weight loss. But in the year 2012, Dr. Michael Mosley, a broadcast journalist of BBC, had popularized intermittent fasting in his TV documentary entitled, "Eat Fast, Live Longer," and his book, "The Fast Diet." After these came out—and gained public interest—a journalist by the name of Kate Harrison launched her own book entitled, "The 5:2 Diet," which was based on her own experiences. Subsequently, Dr. Jason Fung, a nephrologist from Canada, came out with his own bestselling book in 2016 entitled, "The Obesity Code." Soon, intermittent fasting received a constant stream of positive buzz as more and more people started following it and experienced the benefits. Then these people started sharing their stories, which, in turn, helped IF explode in popularity in such a short time.

Before you start following this eating pattern, learning everything that you can about it will help you out immensely. Understanding the science behind IF may help you understand why it works so well. This understanding also makes it easier for you to believe other people when they share their own experiences with IF, whether good or bad. So, in this book, I have combined my own anecdotal experiences along with the stories shared by others I know, plus all of the research I had conducted as I embarked on my own IF journey. To give you a clear picture of what IF is all about and what it does to your body, I will share some of the studies I have read plus sensible advice on nutrition to provide you with everything you need to start fasting intermittently.

When you read about IF, you might think that it's too hard for you to follow. But the truth is, it doesn't have to be. One of the best things about intermittent fasting is that there are many ways to do it. For instance, if you try fasting on alternate days, you may experience the same benefits as trying to fast at specific times each day. If you have never tried fasting before, then fasting for an entire day might be too challenging for you. That's okay because you can ease into IF until you feel more confident about trying the more extreme methods of this eating pattern.

When it comes to following IF, you may have to try different methods before finding the one that is most effective for you. The method you choose should fit your lifestyle, and it must be sustainable for you. Combine this with a healthy diet, and you're sure to find success with intermittent fasting. On the other hand, if you only consume processed or junk foods on IF, you will place yourself at risk for the common dangers and side effects of this diet. This is where the value of research comes in. The more you learn about IF, the more you can prepare yourself for what is to come. Also, you won't have to panic when you start experiencing changes in your body because of the new eating pattern that you follow.

Personally, I do believe in intermittent fasting. In particular, I am a follower of the One Meal A Day or OMAD method. This is one of the more extreme ways, but I didn't start with it right away. My intermittent fasting journey involved trying out different methods until I found the right one. That was when I experienced the benefits that this trendy eating pattern had to offer. Unfortunately, when it comes to OMAD, there aren't a lot of resources that provide comprehensive information about it. I had to do a lot of research just to understand this method, how to follow it correctly, and even the potential risks it comes with. The good news is, after discussing the basics of intermittent fasting, we will be focusing on the

OMAD method to help you determine if it is the right one for you.

WHAT IS INTERMITTENT FASTING?

If you're thinking about the best ways to improve your health, then intermittent fasting might help you out. Intermittent fasting isn't a diet—it's an eating pattern wherein you would cycle between eating and fasting. While diets focus on the quantity and quality of the food you eat, intermittent fasting focuses on when you eat or the timing. This is why the main difference between the various methods of intermittent fasting is the variation in schedules. Later, we will discuss these methods in detail.

As you follow intermittent fasting, you would have "feasting windows" and "fasting windows." During your feasting windows, you allow yourself to eat whatever you want for a certain period of time. Usually, this would last for a specific number of hours. Then when your fasting window starts, you would stop consuming solid foods or beverages that contain calories. However, you can consume non-caloric beverages like water or plain tea and coffee.

If you fast long enough, your insulin levels will go down to the point where your body switches from burning glucose to burning fat. At this point, your body reaches a metabolic state known as "ketosis" wherein it becomes a fat-burning machine.

Another way to look at it is this: when you fast long enough, you starve your body of glucose, its primary source of energy. As soon as your body's glucose stores have been depleted, ketosis kicks in. Then your body turns to your fat stores to keep it functioning. But fat-burning isn't the only benefit of ketosis. In the same way, intermittent fasting also offers a number of health benefits, which we will go through in the next chapter.

While intermittent fasting is a relatively new concept in the sense that it is now being used for weight loss and other health purposes, the actual practice of fasting has been around from the beginning. Many religions and cultures have been fasting as part of their ancient traditions. For instance, Theravada Buddhist monks practice fasting as part of their monastic training. From noon to the time the sun rises on the next day, they practice fasting—and they do this every day. Islam also practices fasting, using a method similar to IF during Ramadan. In the morning, before dawn, they consume a meal to prepare themselves for the fast. From dawn until the sun sets, they don't eat anything. Then in the evening, they allow themselves to eat again. However, they only do this for one month, and it's not part of their normal lifestyle. These are just two of the most common examples of how fasting is utilized as a part of religious practices.

Apart from this, fasting has also been used in a therapeutic way at least since the year 1915. Back then, it was used to help treat people who suffered from obesity. Around the 1960s, the medical community had a renewed interest in fasting. This time, they focused on short-term or intermittent fasts to determine the health benefits these fasts have to offer. Since then, intermittent scientists and researchers have conducted so many studies about IF that when 2012 rolled in, this eating pattern suddenly became all the rage.

Intermittent fasting will only work if you follow it correctly. No matter what method you have chosen, it's essential for you to fast completely during your fasting window. This means no snacks whatsoever, not even a sugary drink with whipped cream on top. If this is your first time fasting, then IF might be a challenge for you. However, the longer you stick with the eating pattern, the more your body will adjust to it. When this happens, then you will find it easier to follow IF. Unlike diets, you won't have to restrict yourself from eating certain foods or eliminate specific food groups from your diet. Of course, it would still be more beneficial for you if you focus on whole foods to ensure that you are getting all the nutrients you need to keep your body healthy.

One factor that would contribute to which method of IF you choose is what your main purpose for following this eating pattern is. Take fat burning, for instance. This is one of the most common reasons why people decide to IF. This also happens to be one of my own reasons for fasting intermittently. To achieve the fat-burning benefit of intermittent fasting, your fasting windows should at least be 12 hours. Then if you can go higher than that, your body may become even more efficient at burning fat. Of course, as a beginner, you would have to work your way up to a fasting window as long as this.

Unlike other diets, fasting doesn't require you to count calories either. It's not a requirement, but it can be beneficial, especially if you want to avoid any health issues like nutrient deficiencies. Take me, for instance, since I follow the OMAD method, I found it more comforting to count the calories of my single meal for the day, especially when I was starting out. After all, I was trying to overcome my insulin resistance, so I made sure that I was doing everything right. Of course, if calorie counting isn't something that you want to do, you don't have to in order to follow IF correctly.

While many of us have found success with IF, this doesn't mean that it's for everyone. Some people have tried following IF but have found it too challenging to sustain. Others have tried too much too fast, which caused them to feel too much pressure. Then there are others who gave up because they didn't see the results or experience the benefits right away. At the end of the day, your success on IF will depend on how committed you are to follow it, how well it can fit into your lifestyle, and if you can follow the method you have chosen correctly. This means that you can only truly determine if intermittent fasting is right for you by trying it out after you have learned all that you can about it.

WHAT HAPPENS TO YOUR BODY WHEN YOU EAT?

Before we discuss what happens to your body while fasting, let me help you understand what happens to your body whenever you eat. In a nutshell, this is what happens: right after eating something, your body starts producing insulin to convert the sugar in the food you ate, the sugar is used to fuel your cells, and whatever is left gets stored in your body as fat. However, these processes won't get triggered when you are following intermittent fasting. Instead, it will result in the activation of other bodily mechanisms.

After eating a meal, the process of digestion follows naturally. Digestion is a process that involves the conversion of food into fuel for the body to absorb and utilize for energy. Digestion can also convert the food you have eaten into raw materials for building or repairing tissues. From head to toe, all of the parts of your body require this energy to keep functioning. All of the organs and systems in your body need fuel to keep functioning. When you eat regularly, the food you eat is the primary energy source of your body.

The digestion process also involves the production of enzymes and acids that mix with the food you eat to break everything down. During this process, the carbohydrate content of your food—the starches and sugars—are broken down into glucose. Then your small intestines and stomach absorb this glucose before releasing it into your bloodstream. After that, the glucose can already be used for energy as needed while any leftover is stored for later use. For your body to start using or storing glucose, it needs the hormone insulin. Without this hormone, glucose remains in your bloodstream, which, in turn, keeps your levels of blood sugar elevated.

The pancreas is the organ in your body that produces insulin. This organ contains beta cells that are highly sensitive to the glucose content in your bloodstream. These beta cells also check your blood glucose levels every couple of seconds so that they can determine whether they need to slow down or speed up the amount of insulin they produce and release. Whenever you eat a high-carb meal, your blood glucose level increases, thus, causing the beta cells in the pancreas to produce and release high amounts of insulin, allowing your body to use or store glucose. After this, your blood glucose levels will start decreasing, thus, causing the beta cells in the pancreas to slow down insulin production.

Throughout the day (and night), this process occurs. The beta cells in your pancreas check your blood glucose regularly. If you are healthy, then your pancreas and beta cells will work normally. The process of utilizing energy and keeping a delicate balance with just the right amount of insulin from the pancreas is essential for your body to maintain the energy it needs to function even while you sleep. However, if you suffer from insulin resistance, this throws your hormone levels off, thus, leading to other issues inside your body. Or if you keep eating throughout the day, especially if you love eating high-carb foods, your body would always need high amounts of insulin. Eventually, your body might not have the capacity to keep up with the amount of food coming in, and your bodily functions start breaking down.

This is where fasting comes in. When you fast, you are giving your body, specifically your digestive system, time to rest, and recuperate. Also, when you don't consume anything, the beta cells in your pancreas won't have to produce insulin since there won't be spikes in your blood glucose levels. Since intermittent fasting involves cycling between periods of eating and fasting, this means that you won't be starving yourself completely. You will eat at some point, but you will be reducing the frequency of your meals so that your body can work more efficiently.

WHAT HAPPENS TO YOUR BODY WHEN YOU FAST INTERMITTENTLY?

Fasting means that you wouldn't consume anything with calories. It's crucial for you to understand the "no calories" part, especially when you start following IF. Just because you're allowed to drink during your fasting windows, this doesn't mean that you can whip up smoothies or blended drinks when you are hungry. Drinking such beverages would break your fast because the sugars and all other calories in these drinks will activate your body's digestive process. If you have been "fasting" this way and you haven't experienced any benefits, those sugary and high-calorie drinks are to blame.

Anyway, going back to fasting... when you stop eating for hours at a time, your body will start working differently. In a nutshell, here are the things that will happen:

- After your body digests the last bit of food from the last meal you ate, it won't be breaking down anything else. Therefore, glucose won't be released into your bloodstream, which, in turn, signals the pancreas to stop producing insulin.
- When there is no more glucose to use, this is when your body turns to the fat stores in your cells for energy.
- With the absence of glucose and insulin, your blood sugar levels stabilize. You won't experience spikes or crashes that tend to make you feel tired or sometimes make you crave certain types of food.
- The longer you fast, the more efficient your body becomes in terms of using energy. This won't happen if you fast intermittently for a week. You may start seeing the benefits if you continue following IF regularly for a couple of months. In the beginning, you may feel tired and have a lack of focus. But when your body starts adjusting, your energy levels will go back up, thus, making you feel better.
- Fasting also gives your digestive system and gut a

much-needed break. It provides a chance to slow down and reset, which, in turn, promotes improvements in the body like a reduction of acid reflux, heartburn, bloating, and other common issues.

As you can see, intermittent fasting works by helping your body learn how to work in a different way. Because of the flexibility of IF, it has become one of the most popular diet trends in the world now. As long as you follow the method or schedule you have chosen consistently and adequately; you can expect to see the benefits of this eating pattern happening after some time.

However, simple as this eating pattern is, it may throw your body "out of whack," especially during the first few days or weeks of your IF journey. This is especially true if you haven't tried fasting before or if you usually eat heavy meals or frequent snacks throughout the day. In such cases, starting on IF means that you would be significantly restricting your food intake. This means that you will feel hungry, and you may experience a number of weird side effects. These are normal... I have experienced some of these too. The important thing is to stick with the eating pattern so that you can give your body time to adjust to it.

Even our earliest ancestors practiced intermittent fasting, although they didn't have a name for it back then. In the past, our ancestors didn't have access to readily-available foods. Therefore, they would only eat when they felt hungry, and before they could eat, they would have to hunt or forage first. If they couldn't find anything, they would be forced to fast. These fasts depended on where and when they would find their next meal. This shows us that back then, snacking wasn't part of their lifestyle. It has only become an extra part of our daily diet since food has become so abundant and readily available to us. Unfortunately, snacking isn't a healthy habit, and it's a definite no-no when you are fasting.

Fasting affects your body in the same way exercise does. When you exercise, your cells experience some level of stress. However, during your workout, those cells don't grow or strengthen—these things happen during the resting or recovery period. In the same way, your cells enter a stress-resistance mode while you fast. It super-charges them so that when you start eating again, they can quickly absorb the nutrients you consume, thus, allowing them to grow and become stronger. This is another way for you to look at how fasting affects your body.

When you start fasting, expect to experience hunger. No matter what method you choose to follow, hunger pangs are one of the most common side effects you will feel, especially when you start fasting intermittently. This is because your body is used to getting a steady supply of glucose from the foods you eat. During your fasting window, your body will feel deprived, which, in turn, causes it to send specific signals that cause hunger pangs. Among all of the side effects you may experience, this is one of the most challenging to deal with. If you focus on your hunger pangs, you won't be able to think of anything else. This, of course, may lead you to convince yourself that it's okay to "just eat something light."

As much as possible, try to resist the urge to give in to your hunger pangs. There are many ways to do this, which we will discuss later. When you stick with your fasting window, your body will adjust to the habit of fasting. This is when your body will learn to use the fat stores in your body for fuel. The longer you remain in your fasting window, the more efficient your body gets at burning fat. Soon, you will notice that your hunger pangs don't happen as frequently as they did in the past. Your appetite will start leveling out, and you will have fewer cravings too.

However, if you feel that, at some point, your hunger pangs are starting to interfere with your life, then you may allow yourself to grab a quick bite. It's never a good idea to restrict yourself so much that you cannot think of anything else. The same thing goes if you start feeling dizzy or lightheaded during your fasting window. Your goal here isn't to starve yourself—it's to train your body to get used to eating less frequently each day. If you can do this without forcing yourself or making yourself feel bad, then you know that you are on the right path.

Now that you know what happens inside your body during your fasting window, you should have a better idea of what to expect when you start on your IF journey. Of course, there are things you can do to make the adjustment more comfortable and ensure your own health and safety. One of the most important things you can do to become successful at IF is to learn how to eat healthily. Although this isn't a requirement while following the eating pattern, it will help you achieve your health goals faster while avoiding the potential pitfalls and risks of IF.

Let's have a moment of reflection here. Try to think of yourself following the intermittent fasting eating pattern right now. Now, imagine that you have chosen to practice the OMAD method after a few months of following one of the easier IF methods. Each day, you would only eat one meal, and this meal would have to keep you full, satisfied, and nourished until the next day. With this in your mind, what kind of meal would you imagine yourself eating? Should it be something quick that you bought from a favorite fast food joint, or should it be something nutrient-dense that you prepared yourself? Should it be a fast-food burger with fries, fried chicken, and a milkshake or a full platter of colorful vegetables, meat, a bowl of soup, and a glass of fresh fruit juice? Between these two options, which do you think will make you feel full and nourished? When you start following IF, you can conduct your own experiments in terms of the food you will eat during your feasting window. This is the best way for you to really experience what will make you feel good and what won't.

As a concept, intermittent fasting has been around since the beginning. As you learn about fasting and its effects on your body, this will, hopefully, make the process less intimidating. After all, you are already fasting right now. From the time you have your last meal of the day to the time you have your first meal of the next day, this is already considered a fasting window. So you can actually plan your fasting window to include this time. It's all about coming up with the best strategy for your body to adjust, especially at the beginning.

IS INTERMITTENT FASTING RIGHT FOR YOU?

What is your main reason for wanting to follow intermittent fasting?

These days, most people give intermittent fasting a try because they want to lose weight. If this is your main reason or one of your reasons, then there is a very high possibility that intermittent fasting can help you out. However, as you may have already realized, IF offers more than just weight loss. This fantastic eating pattern can contribute to the actual improvement of your health, especially if you practice it correctly.

But how do you know that IF is right for you? Well, the best way to find out is to give it a try. In this chapter, you learned what intermittent fasting is and how it affects the body compared to when you eat consistently throughout the day. Of course, all of these things are just explanations to help you understand IF and prepare yourself for what to expect when you start it. Hopefully, everything you have discovered in this chapter has piqued your interest in the diet. Now, all you have to do is to keep exploring the different chapters. In each chapter, you will learn something new about IF until you reach a profound understanding of how you can use it to change your life.

In the pages of this book, I have also shared some of the most effective and practical tips to follow IF that I swear by. Since I started my IF journey with the purpose of overcoming my insulin resistance, I was driven to make it work. I committed to IF, and I learned everything I can to know exactly how I can follow this eating pattern and experience all the benefits it has to offer. You can learn this too and, hopefully, improve your health and your life as much as I have. At this point, the best advice I can give you is to keep moving forward. There is a reason why IF has surged in popularity and gained so many enthusiastic followers. And by learning all about it through this book, you can start your own IF journey and look forward to all the good things it can bring to your life. So, let's keep going!

2

THE MANY HEALTH BENEFITS OF INTERMITTENT FASTING

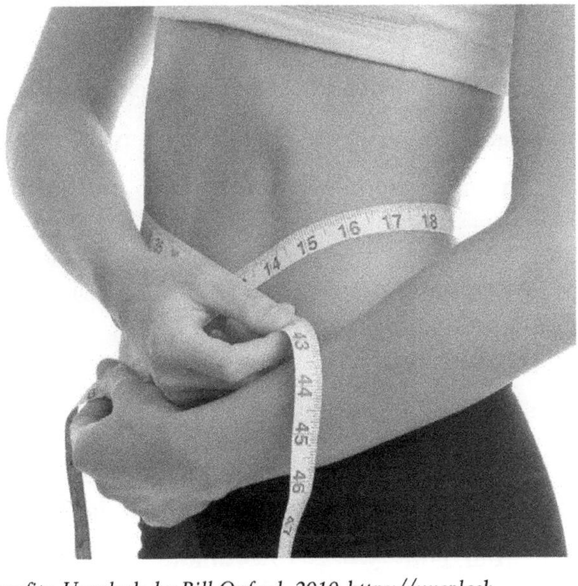

Fig. 3: Benefits. Unsplash, by Bill Oxford, 2019, https://unsplash.com/photos/aIlAhLdwk2g/ Copyright 2019 by Bill Oxford/Unsplash.

According to studies, both animal and human, intermittent fasting offers wide-ranging health benefits. Although more research is needed to solidify all of these claims, the sheer number of anecdotal reports and scientific evidence is already overwhelming enough to encourage people to believe in the potential of this eating pattern. And the fact that fasting has been around for centuries also strengthens the argument for IF, don't you think?

As someone who has done a lot of research on IF and has been following it for a long time now, I can attest to the benefits it has to offer. However, anecdotal reports shouldn't be enough for you. It's also helpful to read the studies and research conducted about IF to help you understand why these benefits exist and why they might not happen for you. This becomes even more important if you want to understand the scientific aspect of the benefits IF has to offer. Therefore, this chapter is dedicated to the benefits of intermittent fasting.

Here, I will share with you the good things that this eating pattern has to offer. I have included some of the most interesting studies I've read through research for you to have a deeper understanding of why this eating pattern changes the way your body works to promote the improvement of your health. Of course, you can also do your own research as you learn about IF. Just make sure that the resources you read offer truthful information. Sadly, there are many sites and written resources that tend to exaggerate the benefits without sharing the other side of the story. Intermittent fasting has a lot of potential benefits, but it also comes with its own risks. Finding out the good and bad sides of IF gives you a better look at the big picture. Later, we will be going through the potential risks to look out for. But for now, let's focus on the scientific and clinical side of the benefits intermittent fasting has to offer.

WEIGHT LOSS

Weight loss is an important benefit of intermittent fasting, although this isn't the only good thing that can come from following this eating plan. Since this is the most common benefit most people look forward to, let's discuss it first. One of the main problems with following a diet is sustainability. In the beginning, you may feel excited and motivated to follow a diet correctly, especially if you start seeing yourself lose weight. But when you get bored of the diet, you become too busy to follow it correctly, or you feel like it has become too challenging (because of the restrictions), then you might go back to your old diet. Often, this may result in regaining all of the weight you lost while on the diet. This is one of the main reasons why a lot of people jump from one diet to another.

This isn't something you would have to worry about with intermittent fasting. Since IF is an eating pattern, you can make it part of your lifestyle. One of the studies I have read confirmed that many people who decide to follow IF do so for the weight loss benefit (Johnstone, 2015). Since you won't be eating throughout the day as you might have been doing in the past IF will reduce the number of meals you eat each day. Furthermore, IF also enhances the functions of your hormones to promote weight loss. Of course, this would only apply if you eat normally during your feeding windows. You don't have to compensate for the meals you've missed by overeating at every meal. If you do this, then weight loss won't be one of the benefits you can expect from IF.

According to a review of the scientific literature of IF, it can cause a person to lose up to 8% of their overall weight over 3 to 24 weeks (Barnosky, et. al., 2014). During fasting, your insulin levels go down while norepinephrine and growth hormone levels go up. These hormonal changes promote fat burning for the body to have fuel to use for energy. Moreover, intermittent fasting can increase your metabolic rate by up to 14% to help your body burn more calories. This means that IF is highly effective for weight loss because it works in two main ways: it reduces your caloric intake and gives your metabolic rate a boost. In the same review conducted in 2014, IF helped the participants lose between 4% to 7% of the circumference of their waists. This means that a lot of the weight they lost came from their belly fat—where fat is typically stored.

Continuing on the topic of weight loss, another great thing about intermittent fasting is that it doesn't cause a lot of muscle loss compared to following a diet where you would have to restrict your caloric intake continuously. In one particular study, the results showed that IF only resulted in 10% muscle loss out of the total weight loss of the participants. Conversely, diets that promote caloric restriction resulted in 25% muscle loss out of the total weight loss (Varady, 2011). The findings of this study suggest that the diets might be as effective as intermittent fasting in terms of weight loss, but you won't have to sacrifice your muscle mass by following IF.

Although there are several other studies that focus on the weight loss aspect of intermittent fasting, these are the simplest to understand, and they provide great explanations for why IF promotes sustainable weight loss. Since this is the most sought-after benefit of the eating pattern, there are factors you can focus on to improve your chances. These factors include your calorie intake, the quality of food that you consume, your consistency, and a lot of patience. These can also promote the other health benefits that IF has to offer.

SLOW DOWN THE AGING PROCESS

The next benefit of IF that I will share with you is the delay of the aging process. Because of the changes that occur inside your body when you fast, this can help prevent or delay the onset of age-related medical conditions too. All methods of intermittent fasting offer this benefit. What's better is that you can enjoy this benefit even if weight loss doesn't come right away. The slowing down of the aging process and the delay of age-related conditions occur because of a process known as "metabolic switching."

The researchers of one particular study discovered the role of this process when it gets activated through intermittent fasting (Anton, et. al., 2017). When you fast, you will starve your body of glucose, which it needs for fuel. Because of this, your body resorts to a different source of energy. When this happens, your liver starts breaking fatty acids down into ketones, which your body then uses for fuel. Since this process stops when your feeding window begins, the process of breaking down fats stops too. But the good news is, intermittent fasting enables metabolic switching wherein your body switches between ketones and glucose, the primary sources of fuel.

According to the researchers, metabolic switching activates a lasting cellular response, which, in turn, provides a protective effect to the body. Alternating between fuel sources through intermittent fasting helps to reduce inflammation, protects your body against the damages of oxidative stress, and boosts your metabolism. All of these are important to prevent the onset of age-related diseases and to keep your body young and healthy. The best part is, these benefits keep coming even after you have gone back to "eating normally."

In another study, the researchers focused on the role of nutrition in preventing age-related disorders (Descamps, et. al., 2005). The results of this study suggest that intermittent fasting can promote an antioxidant effect along with the reduction of oxidative stress that causes aging and the diseases related to it. In particular, the calorie restriction aspect of intermittent fasting is behind this benefit. The restriction of calories by reducing the number of meals you consume each day supports specific mechanisms that promote healthy aging, namely antioxidant effects, autophagy, the proliferation of cells, inflammation, and mitochondrial physiology. All of these mechanisms are related to each other, and they all contribute to the aging benefit of IF.

Naturally, when the aging process slows down, it also lowers the risk of age-related diseases. This, in turn, may even extend your lifespan. Studies conducted on rats have shown that a longer lifespan is another benefit of intermittent fasting. In one of these studies, it showed that IF enhances the survival of mature rats even if they have passed the age at which the growth of their body weight typically comes to a halt (Goodrick, et. al., 1983). In another study that still focused on rats, the researchers discovered that IF helps slow down the rate of aging (Sogawa & Kubo, 2000). The results showed that IF helped increase the maximum lifespan of the rats while inhibiting the development of several age-related conditions. In this study, the rats that followed intermittent fasting lived longer than the rats that were always fully-fed. This also applied to the rats on IF that were heavier than the ones eating throughout the day. Although these studies were conducted on rats, age-related benefits and longevity remain to be well-documented benefits of intermittent fasting.

SAFELY IMPROVE TYPE-2 DIABETES AND METABOLIC SYNDROME

The benefits of intermittent fasting just keep coming as it can also be a safe intervention for the treatment of type-2 diabetes and metabolic syndrome. This easily tolerable eating pattern can help improve these conditions when followed correctly. However, if you suffer from these conditions or any type of medical condition for that matter, it's best to consult with your doctor first. It's not recommended to make any changes to your eating habits without first asking for advice from your personal physician. Your doctor might even offer you valuable advice about how to start fasting intermittently.

Going back to this benefit, let's start with type-2 diabetes. The main feature of this chronic condition is high levels of blood sugar in the context of insulin resistance. Since intermittent fasting helps reduce insulin resistance (this is one benefit that I have experienced firsthand) and helps lower your levels of blood sugar, it can help protect you against this disease. In one study, IF improved the conditions of middle-aged men who suffered from type-2 diabetes (Furmli, et. al., 2017). In this study, the researchers noted that the participants lost weight, they got well enough to stop taking insulin, and they also reduced the oral medication they were taking. According to the researchers, medications might not be as effective for treating this condition as dietary changes are. But when you change your diet, you would be addressing the underlying cause of the condition.

Another study highlighted the benefits of insulin on the improvement of insulin resistance (Barnosky, et. al., 2014). The results of this study showed that the participants showed a significant reduction in their levels of blood sugar. The researchers observed that the fasting blood sugar of participants went down by as much as 6% while their fasting insulin levels went down by as much as 31%. In a different study, the researchers suggested that IF can be a tolerable and safe dietary intervention in patients who suffered from type-2 diabetes (Arnason, et. al., 2017). This effect happens as the eating pattern improves the fasting glucose levels and the bodyweight of the patients. Yet another study supported the same findings as the researchers discovered that IF can help with weight loss, reduce the risk of the disease, and even improve memory (Carter, et. al., 2018).

Unlike type-2 diabetes, metabolic syndrome isn't a single disease. It's an umbrella term used for several risk factors of severe medical conditions like heart disease, stroke, and even diabetes. A recent study focused on the potential role of intermittent fasting in the improvement of metabolic syndrome (Wilkinson, et. al., 2019). This relatively new study looked at the weight loss and health benefits of the eating pattern in rodents and people. The results of this study had shown very promising potential in terms of using intermittent fasting as a lifestyle intervention in the treatment of people suffering from metabolic syndrome. The weight loss benefit of IF can improve the condition, especially when paired with other lifestyle changes like exercise and stress management.

This study involved a rigorous clinical trial where the participants were given a 10-hour feeding window where they had the freedom to eat what they want and when they want. Most of the participants in this study were obese, and more than 80% of them were taking medications. With the conditions set by the researchers, the participants had complete control over their diet within this feeding window, and they even had the opportunity to set the feeding window based on their regular daily schedule. Because of this freedom, the participants felt good about the schedule. As they started following the IF schedule, they started sleeping better and discovered that they had more energy. This prompted them to keep going. The clinical trial ran for three months, and by the end of it, the participants had an average BMI reduction of 3% with a 3% reduction of visceral or abdominal fat. These and all other improvements helped reduce the risk factors of metabolic syndrome. Moreover, the participants were very much willing to continue with intermittent fasting because they felt that it was easy to follow.

SUPPORTS CARDIOVASCULAR HEALTH

Cardiovascular disease is one of the most common causes of death in the world, but just like metabolic syndrome, this isn't a single disease. Cardiovascular disease encompasses different diseases, including hypertension, heart failure, stroke, atrial fibrillation, and so on. There are many risk factors associated with cardiovascular disease. Fortunately, there is evidence that IF has a positive effect on cardiovascular health by stabilizing cholesterol levels, reducing blood pressure, and improving the other risk factors of cardiovascular disease.

One study I have read focused on the weight loss benefit of intermittent fasting for the benefit of cardiovascular health (Varady, et. al., 2009). In this study, the researchers aimed to lower the risk of cardiovascular disease in obese individuals through the eating pattern. The findings of their study showed that intermittent fasting is, indeed, a viable option for those who suffer from obesity to shed their excess pounds and decrease their risk of cardiovascular disease. Another study about cardiovascular health focused on the metabolic effects of intermittent fasting on people who suffer chronic conditions that may lead to cardiovascular disease (de Azevedo, et. al., 2012). The researchers of this study reported that IF has positive effects on the metabolic disturbances caused by chronic conditions, thus, making it an accessible and viable intervention for the improvement of cardiovascular health.

There is some speculation that IF can also change our gut microbiome. The human microbiome consists of collective microorganism genomes. According to experts, these microorganisms are highly dynamic and they go through cyclical fluctuations in terms of their composition each day (Zarrinpar, et. al., 2014). Because of the nature of intermittent fasting and how it changes our metabolism, it can also affect this microbiome in our gut. The most significant effect is the reduction of the cyclical fluctuations that occur daily. This, in turn, can help reset the composition of our microbiome and restore key microbiota to improve all aspects of our health, including our cardiovascular health.

I also came upon a review with the purpose of providing an overview of all the most recent intermittent fasting literature, especially in terms of how it can affect cardiometabolic health (Antoni, et. al., 2014). Here are some highlights of this review:

- In individuals who had a healthy weight, following intermittent fasting for two to three weeks might not have a significant effect on their blood pressure or resting heart rate.
- In terms of gender-specific effects of intermittent fasting over the course of three weeks, changes in the levels of HDL cholesterol were only observed in females. On the other hand, decreases in triglyceride levels were only observed in males.

While many studies have shown promising results, there are a few which suggest inconsistencies such as these. As such, the best course of action is for the experts to continue doing further research on the benefit of IF on cardiovascular health to ease the minds of those who are interested in following the eating pattern to specifically improve their cardiovascular health.

REDUCES THE RISK OF CANCER

By now, you may have noticed that intermittent fasting has a protective effect on the body. This is a very important benefit as it can prevent the development of various diseases, even cancer. Among all diseases, cancer is one of the worst. This terrible disease is mainly characterized by the uncontrolled growth of cancerous cells. If you cannot control this growth through treatment or other kinds of interventions, the disease will just keep getting worse.

Fortunately, intermittent fasting offers a number of metabolic benefits that can help reduce the risk of cancer. There aren't many studies conducted on humans that focus on this benefit. However, there are several animal studies that show promising results in terms of the prevention of this debilitating disease. In one particular study, the researchers found out that fasting may help protect the healthy cells in the bodies of mice from the adverse side effects of the drugs administered during chemotherapy (Lee, et. al., 2012). This effect can potentially apply to humans too. According to the study, multiple fasting cycles can promote the differential sensitization of stress in tumors. This intervention even has the potential to augment or replace the efficacy of specific drugs administered during chemotherapy.

Although the scientific side of this benefit is still in its infancy, the power of intermittent fasting in the prevention or reduction of the risk of cancer lies in its effects on the cells. The general underlying theory of IF in terms of cancer is how it helps our cells adapt to stress. It is believed that healthy cells are more efficient at adapting to a lack of nutrients compared to cancer cells. The latter needs to consume a lot of nutrients to grow. Of course, if you alternate between cycles of eating and fasting, this means that while fasting, you will be starving the cancer cells too. Furthermore, if you are undergoing chemotherapy treatment while following IF, this could increase the susceptibility of the cancer cells to DNA damage and oxidative stress. In other words, IF can potentially make the cancer cells more sensitive to chemotherapy treatment.

More evidence is pointing to the effectiveness of fasting for a period of 18 hours and allowing yourself to eat normally for the remaining 6 hours. According to experts, this might be the ideal ratio for your body to trigger the "metabolic switch" where your body starts burning fat instead of glucose. When your body is in this state, you experience a greater resistance to stress, improved longevity, and a decreased risk of developing various diseases, including cancer. One particular study showed that when obese mice were placed on IF, this reduced the accumulation of fat in their livers, decreased the inflammatory expression of their genes, and reduced their risk of cancer (Varady & Hellerstein, 2007). For this benefit, there have been numerous studies conducted on animals, and here are some highlights of the most interesting ones that I have read:

- One study has indicated that intermittent fasting can help decrease the spontaneous occurrence of tumors in rats (de Cabo & Mattson, 2019).
- Another study has reported that intermittent fasting can help prevent cancer cells from metabolizing energy, thus, hindering their growth and making them more vulnerable to treatments such as chemotherapy (O'Flanagan, et. al., 2017). This same study also suggested that intermittent fasting can help decrease the side effects that may come from certain cytotoxic treatments.

While most studies focused on animals, there was one that focused on the effect of intermittent fasting on people who suffered from breast and ovarian cancer who were undergoing chemotherapy (Bauersfeld, et. al., 2018). This study raised my spirits as it was done on humans, not rats. Here, the participants had to start their fast 36 hours before their chemotherapy session then end it 24 hours after their chemotherapy session. After the trial, the participants who underwent fasting experienced less fatigue, along with an improvement in their quality of life during their chemotherapy sessions. All of these studies are indeed promising, and hopefully, there will be more to provide concrete and consistent evidence on how IF can prevent or improve different types of cancer.

SUPPORTS NEUROLOGICAL HEALTH

Whether this benefit has crossed your mind or not, it is one of the most important benefits of intermittent fasting. If we want to live long, happy, and productive lives, we should also focus on maintaining our neurological health. Intermittent fasting proves to be one of the best diet choices you can make as it can also support the health of the nervous system, enhances cognitive function, and helps reduce the risk of developing neurodegenerative diseases. These benefits come from the restricted eating times that come with intermittent fasting.

Generally, anything that improves the health of your body would also improve the health of your brain. The metabolic benefits of intermittent fasting, such as the reduction of inflammation, oxidative stress, and blood sugar levels, are all important for neurological health. As with all the other benefits, there have been several animal studies conducted that show how intermittent fasting can be beneficial for the brain. For instance, one study has shown that intermittent fasting can help with the process known as neurogenesis—the process by which the neural stem cells produce neurons (Lee, et. al., 2000). This study and similar ones provide valuable insight in terms of how diet can affect the plasticity of the brain to prevent the development of neurodegenerative disorders.

In another study, the researchers discovered that intermittent fasting may promote the production of a brain hormone known as brain-derived neurotrophic factor or BDNF (Mattson, 2005). This is significant since a deficiency of BDNF is associated with different brain issues like depression. An increase in the levels of BDNF in the brain also strengthens neuronal resistance to avoid degeneration and dysfunction. There was also a study related to this brain hormone, but this time, it focused on Huntington's disease (Duan, et. al., 2003). People who suffer from this disease have low levels of BDNF. Since intermittent fasting can help increase the production of this hormone, it can be an excellent dietary intervention for carriers of the mutant huntingtin gene. It can potentially prevent the disease from developing, thus, increasing the lifespan of those who carry the gene.

Intermittent fasting doesn't just protect the brain—it can also improve brain structures and cognitive functions. These were the results of one study done on mice (Liaoliao, et. al., 2013). In a separate animal study, the researchers discovered that intermittent fasting could potentially protect the brain against Alzheimer's disease (Zhang, et. al., 2017). People who suffer from Alzheimer's disease have an excessive accumulation of the protein amyloid-β (Aβ) in their brains. If this accumulation can be avoided or cleared up, it can help prevent or improve the disease. The results of the study showed that intermittent fasting could help prevent the accumulation of Aβ in the brain, thus, preventing the risk of developing the disease. Since intermittent fasting is relatively easy to follow, this can be suggested for the prevention of Alzheimer's disease.

Although fasting has been around for a long time now, scientists and researchers have yet to explore all the potential benefits and applications, especially in terms of the debilitating neurological diseases that plague our world today. But what we do know is that intermittent fasting induces a different kind of metabolic state that improves the resilience, bioenergetics, and plasticity of the neurons in our brains. This fact and all the promising results of the studies that focus on the brain health benefit of intermittent fasting show us that this eating pattern is good for our most important organ. Over time, you may experience improvement in your cognitive skills. Intermittent fasting may even improve the functional recovery of the brain for people who have experienced a brain injury or stroke. Hopefully, we will continue hearing about studies that solidify the claims and make us feel more confident in this benefit of intermittent fasting.

AUTOPHAGY

Autophagy is an essential mechanism in the body wherein the old, damaged, and dead organic materials (like proteins, cell membranes, organelles, and so on) are recycled to repair or create healthy cells. In other words, this is a natural, regulated process that degrades and recycles cellular components. Autophagy is the body's way of clearing out useless materials to create newer and healthier cells. You want this process to happen within your body because it comes with its own host of health benefits. One of the most effective ways to trigger autophagy is through intermittent fasting.

The key activator of this bodily mechanism is nutrient deprivation. Remember that fasting causes your insulin levels to go down, especially when your body has already used up all the glucose from the last meal you consumed. When your body's insulin levels go down, the production of a hormone called glucagon increases. This increase activates the process of autophagy. As this process is activated, you also experience an increase in your growth hormone levels. This means that as autophagy clears out all unnecessary cellular components, your body also works hard to produce new cells. It's like your body is undergoing a much-needed renovation.

One study has shown how nutrient restriction is key to the activation of autophagy (Antunes, et. al., 2018). Since nutrient restriction occurs regularly when you follow intermittent fasting, this means that your body will undergo autophagy regularly too. Here are some benefits this process offers:

- It helps with the regulation of the mitochondria of cells to improve the production of energy.
- It encourages the growth of nerve and brain cells while providing a protective effect on the entire nervous system.

- It encourages the growth of heart cells while protecting you against heart disease.
- It provides a protective effect on DNA stability.
- It gives your immune system a boost by getting rid of intracellular pathogens.
- It prevents healthy organs and tissues from getting damaged.
- It has the potential to combat neurodegenerative diseases, cancer, and other types of illnesses.

Fasting increases the rate of apoptosis (cell death) along with autophagy. This is another natural process that helps to improve our health. After the cells die, autophagy starts recycling the components of those cells. Then comes the renewal of cells and even the production of new cells. Of course, the longer your fasting period is, the longer these processes can continue working. However, as soon as you eat something, these processes all come to a halt.

There was one study done that revealed an important aspect of this process (Mihaylova, et. al., 2018). Here, the researchers discovered the oxidation of fatty acids inside the cells' mitochondria actually improves the function of our stem cells. This is a very important benefit since our stem cells tend to lose their efficiency as we age. Since autophagy can help renew these cells and intermittent fasting activates this metabolic process, this means that autophagy also has a positive impact on aging and our overall health.

Of course, this is just one study. But one thing is for sure—autophagy is an essential process in the body to keep you young, renewed, and healthy. There is a lot more to this process for you to learn about, and you can do this by going online and doing research about it. I have shared with you the basics of autophagy and how it can benefit the body in relation to intermittent fasting. But being a complex process in itself, you can understand it better by learning more about it. What I can say for now is that intermittent fasting is an important stimulator of autophagy. This, in turn, also allows you to enjoy all of the benefits autophagy has to offer.

OTHER HEALTH BENEFITS

I could go on and on about the benefits of intermittent fasting. But I have already shared the most significant ones, and with this last point, I will go through a few others. Intermittent fasting is wonderful as it stimulates a number of changes in the body to optimize the way it works. Here are some other benefits that could be linked to intermittent fasting according to various studies:

Reduces Inflammation

This benefit of intermittent fasting can help in the prevention or management of pro-inflammatory conditions. Although IF provides this benefit, it doesn't have a negative effect on the response of the immune system to acute infections. Caloric restriction has pro-inflammatory effects, as shown in one study (Jordan, et. al., 2019). Although the results of this study have shown that intermittent fasting can reduce inflammation, the mechanisms by which this occurs aren't completely understood yet. What the researchers know for sure is that the reduction of inflammation can help improve chronic inflammatory diseases. The results of this study were supported by an older study that also showed how intermittent fasting could combat inflammation (Johnson, et. al., 2007). In this older study, the researchers focused on how this benefit can improve our quality of life since inflammation is one of the major causes of different types of diseases and disorders.

Reduces Oxidative Damage

This benefit comes from the process of autophagy. When intermittent fasting stimulates autophagy, the process then repairs your cells to improve cell survival. There are many factors that cause oxidative damage, but when your cells are strengthened, this increases their ability to resist oxidative stress and damage more effectively. Just like inflammation, oxidative stress is one of the risk factors of several chronic diseases. Fortunately, several studies have shown how intermittent fasting may increase your body's oxidative stress resistance (Mattson & Wan, 2004). In another study that focused on aging mechanisms, the researchers suggested that caloric restriction can prolong one's lifespan (Weindruch & Sohal, 2010). This also happens when our cells and our whole body becomes stronger and more resistant to oxidative damage. When you restrict calories through intermittent fasting, different processes kick in, all of which work together to improve your health.

Potentially Improves Aerobic Capacity

Finally, intermittent fasting can also be beneficial to athletes and to those who lead an active lifestyle. For instance, when you choose the alternate-day fasting method, this can increase your endurance and your aerobic capacity since your body will switch to fat-burning instead of glucose-burning. This benefit on endurance is what the researchers observed in mice after they put the mice on the diet for a specific period of time (Marosi, et. al., 2018). The results of this study suggest that fasting intermittently can help rats (and potentially, even humans) reach optimum performance while maintaining good health. The researchers also encouraged further study to prove this fact.

Another study conducted on mice also showed how intermittent fasting helped improve their aerobic capacity (Chaix, et. al., 2014). Here, the mice that followed IF were able to run 60 minutes longer than mice that had access to food all day even though they approximately weighed the same. Then there is the weight loss benefit of intermittent fasting to consider along with the fact that this eating pattern doesn't promote muscle loss. All of these factors contribute to the potential improvement of aerobic capacity.

As you can see, intermittent fasting offers so many significant benefits to your health. Even if you just wanted to shed some excess pounds, you will also see an improvement in your overall health as you continue to stick with this eating pattern. One important thing that you can take away from this chapter is that IF has a lot of potential benefits. Even though most of the studies I have presented were conducted on animals, they have shown incredibly promising results. In the near future, we might hear about human studies that show similar or even better results. As you follow IF, keep an eye on updates in terms of the benefits so that you can use these as one of your motivations to keep going.

3

THE MOST POPULAR WAYS TO DO INTERMITTENT FASTING

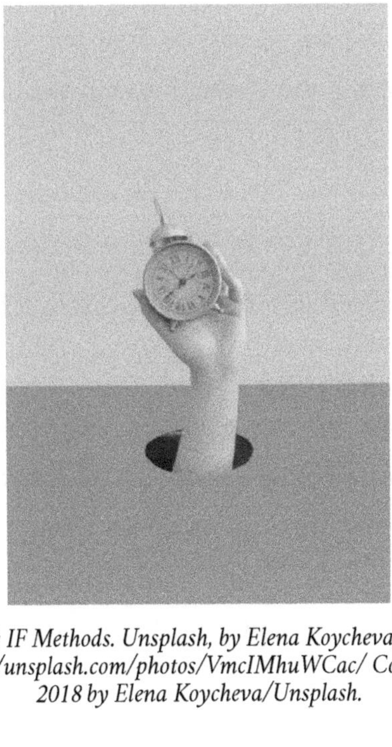

Fig. 4: IF Methods. Unsplash, by Elena Koycheva, 2018, https://unsplash.com/photos/VmcIMhuWCac/ Copyright 2018 by Elena Koycheva/Unsplash.

These days, fasting isn't just done for religious purposes or as part of a tradition. Today, people fast so that they can lose weight, improve their health or even as part of their treatment. Intermittent fasting has become a huge trend in recent years. All around the world, people have been following this eating pattern and because of its effectiveness, the same people have also been singing its praises. Intermittent fasting isn't a diet. It is more of an eating pattern where you would cycle between periods of fasting and eating.

The length and time that these periods happen would depend on the IF method you have chosen. There are several methods of intermittent fasting to choose from but the ones we will discuss here are the most common and popular ones. If it is your first time fasting intermittently, you can start with one of the easier methods and build up gradually to the more intense ones as your body adjusts to intermittent fasting. You can also give the different methods a try to see which one you can follow long-term.

One of the things that I love about intermittent fasting is its flexibility. Even if you have chosen a certain method, you can still customize it to fit into your schedule. This is also one reason why I found it quite easy to adjust to intermittent fasting. The first time I followed it, I made sure that my fasting window included my sleeping time. That way, I had seven to eight hours each day where I didn't have to feel hungry or think about how many hours were left until my next feeding window.

Of course, there were still times when I felt like I wanted to give in to my hunger and once in a while, I did. I indulged in a light snack whenever I felt like I couldn't focus on anything else or when I felt too lightheaded to function. Although allowing myself to give in to my hunger once in a while made me feel bad, I still tried to forgive myself to make things easier. If you're like me and it's your first time fasting, then you might experience challenges similar to this. But if you have had experience with fasting, then your journey might be smoother and easier.

For you to start your intermittent fasting journey, you must first decide which method to follow. To do this, it's recommended that you learn everything you can about the different methods. That way, you can try to determine which one might fit into your lifestyle best and give it a try. Try to pick at least two or three options so that you can shift to a new method if you think that the first one you have chosen isn't working for you. Now, let's go through the different methods to give you a better idea of what your options are.

5:2 METHOD

This is the most common intermittent fasting method. This IF method is also known as the Fast Diet and it was made popular by Michael Mosley, the British journalist. In a nutshell, this method involves fasting twice a week then eating normally for the rest of the days. This is a very flexible method because you can choose which days you will fast and which days you will eat normally. The only rule you would have to follow when you choose this method is that there should be at least one non-fasting day between your fasting days. In other words, this means that you shouldn't fast for two days straight.

During your fasting days, you would only consume a maximum of 500 calories. Although counting calories isn't a requirement on IF, this practice may help increase your chances of success, especially during your fasting windows. Over time, you will get a good sense of what a 500-calorie meal looks or feels like once you eat it. But in the beginning, counting calories can be very helpful. So if you should only be eating 500 calories on your fasting days, here are some examples of ways to plan to eat your meals:

- You can have a 200-calorie beef cheeseburger with the works (and the bun) in the morning and a 300-calorie hearty winter soup in the afternoon.
- You can start your day with a 300-calorie stir-fry rice bowl with shrimp or chicken then have a lighter 200-calorie meal of fajitas later in the afternoon.
- You can also stick with your 3-meals-a-day plan where you would eat 200-calorie turkey tacos for breakfast, 200-calorie baked tilapia with vegetables for lunch, and a 100-calorie salad for dinner.

As long as you stick with the 500 calories on your fasting days, choosing when to consume your meals is entirely up to you.

However, if you're following this method, it might not be the best option to eat a single 500-calorie meal for your fasting days, especially when you're still starting out. On the days when you aren't fasting, you should eat normally. If you can reduce the number of times you eat—like if you avoid snacking if you don't feel hungry—this might make your fasting days a lot easier. Just make sure that you don't eat more than what you normally do while convincing yourself that it's okay because, on your fasting days, you will be reducing your caloric intake.

Many people believe that this is the easiest IF method to follow. After all, you would only have to fast for 2 days each week and on those days, you won't have to fast completely. You can eat up to 500 calories on those days and you can choose how to spread out your meals. Of course, this method would be much more effective if you choose healthy meals, especially during your fasting days.

The 5:2 method might seem simple and easy, but when you're starting out, you will definitely feel the difference. This is especially true if you are used to eating more than the recommended number of calories each day. This is why you should plan your meals well throughout the day. This is also why it's important to drink regularly to keep yourself hydrated so you won't feel the intensity of your hunger pangs. Also, if you work out, play sports or have high-intensity training sessions, make sure that these strenuous activities don't fall on your fasting days. Otherwise, you might fall ill or even experience the other potential side effects of intermittent fasting. Choose your fasting days wisely to make it easier for you to follow this method.

16:8 METHOD

For this method, you would be fasting daily. Your feasting window would range between 14 to 16 hours giving you a feeding window between eight to ten hours. As with the 5:2 method, you decide when to schedule your fasting windows and feeding windows. Also, you can decide how many meals you want to eat within your feeding window. You can have two large meals, three smaller meals or even four light meals throughout your feeding window. One of the easiest ways to start on this method is by skipping your first or last meal of the day. Let me share an example of how you would create a schedule for following this IF method:

- You can skip breakfast so that your feeding window starts at 10:00 in the morning.
- Let's say that you plan to eat three meals throughout the day. This means that your first meal would be at 10:00 am.
- Your second meal could be around 1:00 or 2:00 in the afternoon.
- Your final meal would be at around 5:00 or 5:30 in the afternoon.
- At 6:00 in the evening, your fasting window begins

and it will end at 10:00 in the morning of the next day.

It looks simple, doesn't it? The 16:8 method is another easy IF method to follow and it's recommended for beginners. If you don't think that you can fast for 16 hours a day, then you can opt for the 14:10 method—a variation of this method. The 14:10 method may be more realistic and easier for you to follow because you would have an extra two hours for your feeding window. Using the same example as above, your day might look like this:

- You can skip breakfast so that your feeding window starts at 9:00 in the morning.
- Since your feeding time has been extended, you can plan to eat four meals throughout the day. This means that your first meal would be at 9:00 am.
- Your second meal could be around 12:00 noon.
- Then you can have a light snack around 3:00 in the afternoon.
- Your final meal would be at around 6:00 or 6:30 in the afternoon.
- At 7:00 in the evening, your fasting window begins and it will end at 9:00 in the morning of the next day.

Of course, if you're an early bird, you can start your feeding window at an earlier time. The key here is to eat what you want and need to within your feeding window, whether you choose eight or ten hours. If you have a day job, you can choose to set your feeding window at the same time as your working hours. That way, you will have the energy to work productively throughout the day. And when you go home, all you have to do is relax, wind down, and go to sleep.

Since this method involves fasting every day, it may take some time for you to find the perfect schedule. For instance, if you decide to set your feeding window at the same time as your working hours, you might discover that you're too busy to have time to eat. When this happens, your fasting window might end up being too long. In such a case, then you might have to move your feeding window to a different schedule—one where you can guarantee that you can eat enough to stay healthy each day. This method is relatively simple and it's not as extreme as the others. Therefore, you can try it out even if you have no prior fasting experience.

ALTERNATE-DAY FASTING METHOD

This method is like a different version of the 5:2 method. Instead of setting fasting and feeding windows for yourself, you would fast on alternate days. This means that every other day, you would eat regularly. Then on the days in between, you would have a fasting day wherein you restrict your caloric intake. To follow this method, you won't fast completely on your fasting days. Instead, you will reduce your caloric intake significantly—by around 70% to 75%. For instance, if your normal caloric intake for the day is 1,800 calories (on your normal eating days), then you would reduce this to 450 calories on your fasting days. Let me share an example of how your week would go as you start following this method:

- On Monday, you consume your normal 1,800 calories throughout the day.
- On Tuesday, you aim for only 450 calories. You can have a heavy 300-calorie meal in the morning and a lighter 150-calorie meal in the afternoon or early in the evening.
- On Wednesday, you go back to consuming your normal 1,800 calories throughout the day.
- On Thursday, you go back to 450 calories. You can have a light breakfast, lunch, and dinner wherein each meal only contains 150 calories.
- On Friday, you consume 1,800 calories spread throughout your day.
- On Saturday, you limit yourself to 450 calories again. This time, you can have a light 200-calorie meal in the morning and the evening with an even lighter 50-calorie snack in between.
- On Sunday, you go back to your normal 1,800 calories.

For the next week, you would switch the schedule as Monday becomes a fasting day. You can continue alternating between normal and fasting days if it works for you. You may have noticed that I provided different options for your fasting days. You can do this too. Find out what works best for you by trying out different things. If you think that consuming two meals on your fasting days is enough, stick with it. If not, then you can try a different approach.

For some people, this method is too difficult to follow. Usually, they are referring to the more advanced version of this method wherein fasting days are days when you literally fast, thus consuming zero calories. Throughout the day, you only drink water and other non-caloric drinks. As a beginner, I don't recommend this for you. Even if you have experience with fasting in the past, doing it every other day one week after another isn't recommended. Remember that fasting changes the way your body works. Although these changes can lead to a lot of health benefits, shocking your body by trying to fast for long periods of time and too frequently, you might end up compromising your health.

If you want to move forward with IF, it's best to start off slow. For instance, you can start with this method by just restricting your caloric intake on fasting days. When your body has adjusted to the caloric restriction, then you can reduce your food intake on your normal days by just a bit. For instance, if you normally consume 1,800 calories, you can bring this down to 1,600 calories. Follow this eating pattern for about a month or so to give your body time to adjust. Then you can try reducing your caloric intake on your fasting days. For instance, instead of consuming 450 calories, you can bring this down to 350 or 400 calories.

You need to go through a process of adjustment if you want to get the best results and if you want this eating pattern to work for you. These small modifications help your body adjust to intermittent fasting more effectively, thus, making the eating pattern more sustainable for you. You also have the choice to start with a different method and shift to the more advanced version of this one. The flexibility of IF means that you can try different methods until you find the method (and the variation) that suits your own lifestyle.

EAT-STOP-EAT METHOD

This method is one of the more intense ones, thus making it more challenging. Although I don't recommend it for you if you're an IF beginner, it's still worth learning about in case you will shift into this method in the future. This method is also known as the 24-hour fast because it involves fasting for one whole day. Typically, you would perform these 24-hour fasts once or twice each week. So the name of this method is quite literal as you will eat for a few days, stop for a day, eat again, and stop... eat-stop-eat.

This method is considered more difficult because it involves a full 24-hour period of not consuming anything at all. To keep your hunger at bay, you can only consume plain coffee, plain tea, water, and any other zero-calorie beverages you can find. As with the 5:2 method, you should have a non-fasting day between your 24-hour fasts. Going for two whole days without eating anything could lead to a number of adverse effects, therefore, this isn't recommended. For this method, let me give you an example of how your typical week would go:

- On Monday, you eat normally and dinner would be your last meal.
- On Tuesday, you have breakfast at 8:00 in the morning and nothing else. This is when your fast starts. For the rest of the day, you won't eat anything.
- On Wednesday, you end your fast by having breakfast at 9:00 in the morning to complete the 24-hour fast. Then you eat normally for the rest of the day.
- On Thursday, you again eat normally throughout the day.
- On Friday, you still continue eating normally throughout the day.
- On Saturday, you have breakfast at 8:00 in the morning then start your second 24-hour fast of the week. This means that you won't eat anything for the rest of the day.
- On Sunday, you have breakfast around 9:00 to end

your fast. Then you continue eating normally for the rest of the day.

This is just an example of how you can schedule your fasting days. Here, the fasting days are on Tuesday and Saturday. You can also choose the time when you start your fasting day. For instance, your last meal can be at lunchtime on your fasting day and this would continue until lunchtime the next day. Plan your schedule accordingly so that it becomes easier for you to follow. As with the other methods, it's best to set your fasting days when you know that your schedule won't be too busy and you won't have to perform any strenuous activities.

Since this method is similar to the 5:2 method, it can be the next step you take after following 5:2 for a couple of weeks or months. If you follow the 5:2 method, your body would eventually get used to eating fewer calories for two days each week. Then you can start reducing the number of calories on these days until you can eliminate all calories completely. This is just a suggestion for how you can advance from one method to another. At the end of the day, the decision still lies with you. For instance, if you try following this method for a few weeks and you notice some negative side effects (we'll discuss these later), then you might want to try a method that isn't as extreme.

Of course, if you think that you are ready for 24-hour fasts, you can try them out. If this method makes you feel better or you think that it's helping you reach your health and fitness goals, good for you! Just make sure that your body can sustain this eating pattern without increasing your risk of developing nutrient deficiencies, headaches, and other health issues.

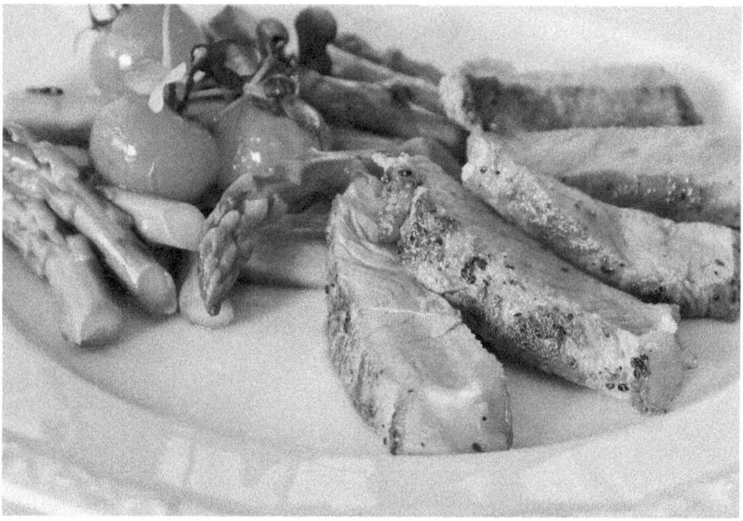

Fig. 5: OMAD. Pixabay, by RitaE, 2017, https://pixabay.com/photos/asparagus-steak-veal-steak-veal-2169305/ Copyright 2017 by RitaE/Pixabay.

ONE MEAL A DAY METHOD

This method is the one that I am following now, and it also happens to be the main focus of this book. The name is pretty self-explanatory as this method involves eating only one meal each day. It's the perfect method for those who lead busy lifestyles or for those who want to give the more extreme methods of intermittent fasting a try. One thing I can tell you right now is that this isn't a method for beginners. Since you will be only eating a single meal each day, you have to plan your meal well.

For a lot of people, they can only eat so much in a single sitting. But if you only eat a "regular meal" like two pieces of chicken, a serving of mashed potatoes, and a glass of juice for the day, you'll definitely feel intense hunger pangs. Also, eating only one small meal every day could lead to nutrient deficiencies, so you should approach this method with enough practical knowledge and a lot of caution.

This method is sometimes called the 23:1 method as it involves 23 hours of fasting and only 1 hour of eating. But the truth is, you can take as long as you want to eat your meal as long as you eat it in a single sitting. If you're in a rush, you might even finish your meal in less than an hour. After your one meal of the day, you can only consume zero-calorie beverages for the rest of the day. If you're like me, you can start following this diet by counting calories. I did this because I wanted to make sure that I wasn't depriving myself. But again, this isn't a requirement. Many people believe that this is the simplest method to follow because all you have to do is eat a single meal each day. As long as the meal you have eaten makes you feel full and satisfied, then it has served its purpose.

Among all the methods of intermittent fasting, this is the one that involves the most caloric restriction in terms of quantity and consistency. No matter how hungry you are, you can only eat so much in a single sitting. So it's quite a challenge to overeat when following this method. Because of this caloric restriction, this method can result in sustainable weight loss along with all of the other benefits linked to intermittent fasting. Personally, I did lose a lot of weight when I started on OMAD. Although I already lost a significant amount of weight when I began my intermittent fasting diet, I did shed even more weight through this method.

One of the first tips I will share with you about OMAD is to focus on healthy foods. Since you will only be eating one meal, make sure it counts. Imagine what would happen to your body if your single meal of the day would always be something greasy, processed or high in sugar. Eating food like this every day and nothing else won't lead to health improvements, but the opposite. If you have already been following IF for some time now and you're ready to switch to OMAD, I will be sharing tips and strategies to help you succeed. The same thing goes for if you're planning to shift to OMAD after allowing your body to adjust to intermittent fasting through one of the easier methods first. When you're ready to start the OMAD routine, then you can apply everything that you will learn in the remaining chapters of this book. But before that, let me share with you the last method that you can start off with.

SPONTANEOUS MEAL SKIPPING METHOD

This final method I will share with you isn't technically considered a method of IF. But for someone who has never tried fasting before, this is the easiest and most relaxed way to start experiencing intermittent fasting. For this method, you would spontaneously skip meals whenever you feel like it. For instance, if you're too busy at work, you decide to skip lunch. Or dinnertime comes, and you're not hungry, you decide to skip dinner and do something else instead. Each time you skip one of your regular meals, this allows you to engage in a certain fasting period. Let me share a more specific example for you:

- In the morning, you start your day with a healthy breakfast.
- Come lunchtime, you have a lot of things to do at work, so you decide to grab a light salad for a quick lunch.
- At around 4:00 in the afternoon, you feel hungry, so you eat a burrito as a snack.
- When it's time for dinner, you still feel full from the burrito you ate, so you decide to have a glass of water before starting your bedtime routine.
- You go to bed and the next morning, you have breakfast at 7:00.

This is a perfect example of spontaneous meal skipping. In this example, the last meal you had was your snack at 4:00 in the afternoon. This means that you would have fasted from around 5:00 in the afternoon to 7:00 in the morning the next day. Although it may have been a spontaneous decision to skip your last meal of the day, you would have already given yourself a fasting window of 14 hours!

For beginners, this is an excellent method because you don't have to follow a strict or structured nutritional regimen. It will just be like giving yourself a chance to practice fasting intermittently without making any commitments yet. Then when you feel like you have gotten the hang of fasting, you can choose one of the IF methods that have flexible rules.

This is also a great option if you eat instinctively. If you're used to eating only when you feel hungry, this method allows you to skip meals whenever you don't feel hungry. If you had already been doing this in the past, that means that you were already following IF on some level. Now, it might be the right time for you to give the other methods a try. Meal skipping is a great way to start your IF journey, but at some point, you should try to make your fasting windows more of a regular thing. That way, you will really train your body to learn how to survive without eating anything for certain periods of time.

As you can see, all of the IF methods are simple and easy to follow. They offer flexibility in terms of when you set the time or day of your fasting window. At this point, you should already have a good idea of which methods can potentially be the ones you choose for your IF journey. Since this book is all about the OMAD method, we will be going into more detail about it in the next chapter. Whether you have chosen this method to follow or you want to try the other methods too, the tips you will learn in the next chapters will also be very helpful for you. So, keep turning those pages!

4

ONE MEAL A DAY METHOD OF INTERMITTENT FASTING

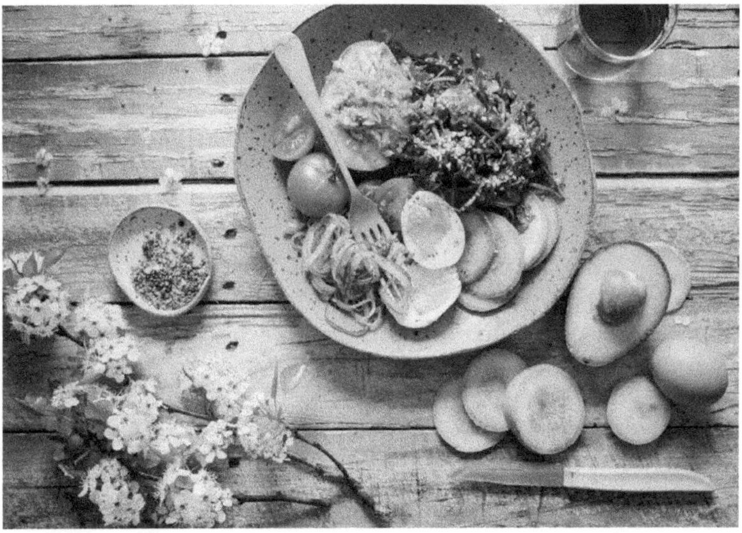

Fig. 6: All About OMAD. Unsplash, by Brooke Larke, 2017, https://unsplash.com/photos/jUPOXXRNdcA/ Copyright 2017 by Brooke Larke/Unsplash.

The One Meal A Day method of intermittent fasting is considered as one of the most extreme methods. But it also happens to be one of the most popular IF methods, especially for those who want to get stellar results in a short amount of time. As I have mentioned in the last chapter, this method is more challenging than the others, especially if you're an IF beginner or if you have never tried fasting before. Still, having been a follower of this diet for quite some time now, I can tell you that there are things you can do to make your OMAD intermittent fasting journey a lot easier.

If your main goal is to lose a lot of weight, OMAD is one of the best methods for you. Of course, this isn't the only benefit you will get from following OMAD. You can look forward to all the other benefits of IF through this method too. But following it entails some education and planning, especially if it's your first time and you want to succeed. As the name implies, you will only eat a single meal each day on OMAD. The flexibility of intermittent fasting comes in the form of the time when you eat your single meal. For instance, if you eat a big, satisfying breakfast, then you won't consume anything until the next day.

It's important to note that "one meal" in this method doesn't mean that you should eat a regular meal. For instance, if your normal meal consists of a scoop of mashed potatoes, a piece of roasted chicken, and a side of buttered veggies, this can tide you over until your next meal. However, if you're on OMAD, you may want to increase your caloric intake a bit. Remember—the single meal you eat should be enough to make you feel full and satisfied. Although it's not recommended to strive to overeat for your one meal of the day, it's also not recommended to pair this method with severe caloric restriction. Fasting is different from starving and you shouldn't aim for the latter.

As a proponent of the OMAD method, I can tell you how it has made my life a lot simpler and easier. I only have to worry about eating one meal a day, but I always make sure that it makes me feel full, satisfied, and happy. I take my one meal at dinner so that I have time to prepare the ingredients for it, cook the dish, and enjoy eating it. After my meal, I relax, wind down, and get ready for bed. No matter how busy I am in the day, no matter how stressful my day has been, this single meal (and the routine that goes with it) makes my days complete. Although I tried following other methods in the past, when I started on OMAD, I realized that I had found the method that was perfect for my own lifestyle. From this chapter, you will learn everything that there is to know about OMAD, and you will have a better idea if this could be the perfect method for you too.

WHY IS OMAD CONSIDERED THE BEST METHOD OF INTERMITTENT FASTING?

When those who know all about IF hear that you follow the OMAD method, they'll think you're hardcore. This is because most people won't purposely choose to only eat one meal for the whole day, every day. However, there is historic evidence that suggests that this method of eating has been around for centuries. Some records even suggest that the Romans only consumed one meal each day. For them, digestion was such an important bodily process that they considered eating more than once each day to be a form of gluttony. For a long time, this belief had an influence on their eating patterns.

In other parts of Europe back in the middle ages, breakfast wasn't considered part of their day. Although most people believe that this is the most important part of the day, even the monarchs in Europe rarely ate this morning meal. Instead, the people in those times had their first meal of the day late in the morning—around 10:00 am or 11:00 am—then have their second meal a few hours later. In the past, people didn't eat as frequently as most people eat now. Back then, this type of eating was a normal part of their lives.

Now, OMAD is making a comeback as more and more people are getting interested in following this extreme yet effective eating pattern. Of course, OMAD isn't a perfect diet nor is it a diet that's suitable for everyone. Because of the nature of this method, you must first think carefully about your current health and eating patterns so that you can determine whether it would be right for you. But, despite all of the potential risks, it still remains to be one of the emerging methods of IF that is gaining more followers. We have already discussed the general benefits of intermittent fasting in Chapter 2. Now, let's take a look at some reasons why the OMAD method is considered to be the best:

Simplicity and convenience

This is the main benefit of OMAD and the reason why I love this eating pattern too. Once you get used to this method, you will discover that it involves minimal planning and preparation. Think about it: how much time do you need for meal planning when you eat three times a day? You have to think of fifteen different meals to prepare for the week for a five-day work-week. On OMAD, all you have to plan for is one meal each day. That reduces the meals you have to plan to only five each week, thus, cutting down your planning time significantly. This covers the convenient aspect of OMAD.

OMAD is also simple—just eat one meal a day. Then all you have to think about is what other things you can do for the day to make yourself as productive as possible. Just don't forget to hydrate yourself throughout the day to avoid any adverse side effects.

More intense health benefits

Since OMAD is an IF method, it means that it also offers the same general benefits as the other methods. But since this is a more advanced and intense method, you can also expect to experience more intense health benefits. Here are some examples:

- You may lose weight faster compared to other IF methods.
- Your human growth hormone levels increase, thus, allowing your body to burn fat while building muscle.
- Your inflammation levels may go down significantly along with your risk of developing certain diseases.
- You may experience an increase in autophagy, which, in turn, offers its own benefits.
- You may experience an improvement in your body's nutritional ketosis, which, in turn, comes with more fat-burning and anti-inflammatory benefits.

Basically, the OMAD method allows you to enjoy the benefits of intermittent fasting more intensely and at a faster rate. Since you will be fasting for longer periods of time each day, you can start feeling the benefits of IF sooner.

If you choose to follow the OMAD diet, try controlling your cravings. Resist your urge to scarf down anything and everything that you crave as soon as it's time for you to eat your one meal of the day. Instead, it's best to opt for healthy, whole foods as these will make you feel more full and more satisfied. Over time, you may notice that you aren't craving unhealthy foods as much as you did in the past. Eating healthily is a choice and the best time to make this choice is when you choose to follow the OMAD method.

THE BENEFITS OF THE OMAD METHOD

As simple as the OMAD method is, it can be quite challenging to follow, especially for first-timers. But with patience, commitment, and consistency, following this diet is entirely achievable. But if you're still on the fence about this extreme method, you may want to learn more about all the benefits it has to offer. OMAD gives you a chance to enjoy all of the benefits that IF has to offer simply because it is an IF method. But there are certain benefits that come with this method exclusively. Let's go through these now:

Fast and effective weight loss

Weight loss is the most sought-after benefit of intermittent fasting. Although this benefit can potentially come from all of the IF methods, you may experience it faster on OMAD. When you only eat a single meal each day, you will definitely be restricting your caloric intake. The great thing about the OMAD method is that it's quite challenging to overeat. For instance, if you have a feeding window of eight hours, you might feel tempted to eat frequently throughout that time. Convincing yourself that it's okay to eat a lot is much easier with a longer feeding window as you would tell yourself that your fasting window is longer anyway. But if you eat more calories than what you normally eat when you're not fasting, you might not see those excess pounds dropping off anytime soon.

On the other hand, when you're on OMAD, you have a maximum of one hour to eat your meal. For a single meal, this is already a lot of time. Usually, eating one satisfying meal will be enough for you, and when your hour is up, it's time for you to start fasting. Even if you use the whole hour to eat, there is a very small likelihood that you can consume all the calories you eat on a regular day at that time. If you do, you might end up feeling sick after!

Because of the very nature of the OMAD method, you will definitely be restricting your caloric intake—and you will do this every day. Naturally, this will cause you to lose weight. This fact was supported by the results of one study where the researchers discovered that the weight loss in people who fasted and people who restricted their overall caloric intake lost was almost the same (Templeman, et. al., 2019). Since OMAD involves fasting and caloric restriction, weight loss will come faster.

When it comes to weight loss sustainability, OMAD shines too. OMAD offers consistency in terms of the method by which you follow the diet. When you train yourself to eat just one meal a day, it becomes easier for your body to adjust. Since the other methods don't offer consistency, it might take more time for your body to adjust to the feeling of fasting. Even if you follow the other methods consistently (which is very important), OMAD is actually easier to adjust to because you will be doing the same thing every day. It's even better if you set your feeding window at the same time each day so you can make it part of your daily routine. When your body adjusts to the eating pattern, you feel more motivated to stick with it. This means that you will continue losing weight until you have reached your healthy weight and maintain it. This benefit was supported by a study wherein the researchers discovered that the participants were able to maintain their weight throughout the study's research period of 6 months (Stote, et. al., 2007). The study also showed that the participants who followed OMAD experienced a reduction in their fat mass. While losing weight is a general benefit of intermittent fasting, OMAD has the potential to improve this benefit compared to the other IF methods.

Better concentration and focus

Following OMAD can do wonders for your concentration and focus. This happens in two ways. First, because of the simplicity of this eating pattern, you don't have to think about where you will have your next meal, what you will eat, or how to budget your food allowance. After planning your one meal of the day, you have all the time to focus on other tasks.

You will feel these benefits, even more, when your body adjusts to the OMAD method. Your body achieves homeostasis once again. After the initial fatigue or weakness, you might experience at the beginning, and your energy levels will start going up. Then you will feel more focused no matter what you are doing, which, in turn, helps you concentrate better. And when it's time for you to have your meal of the day, you can focus on eating too. This makes the experience more satisfying.

Freedom from having to plan several meals throughout the day

This is the best benefit of OMAD for people who lead busy lives. Having to only plan a single meal each day is a relief. Even if you're used to meal planning, all you have to do is think about one meal each day. Shopping and cooking become easier too. And you don't have to resort to eating takeout frequently because you don't have time to prepare your meals. You can always ensure that what you are eating is healthy and nourishing.

You don't need to adhere to strict calorie restrictions

While it's not recommended to overeat while on OMAD, you don't have to restrict your caloric intake either. In fact, it's not recommended to restrict your caloric intake while following this method because you might end up developing nutrient deficiencies. Calorie restriction is the most difficult aspect of a diet. On OMAD, you won't feel like you are restricting yourself, especially if you make sure that your meal always makes you feel full and satisfied.

It might even help improve your performance

When you think of this method, you might not think that it would be suitable for those who live active lifestyles. But the fact is, there are some professional athletes who have started following OMAD to gain all the benefits. One such athlete is

Herschel Walker, the NFL star. He skips breakfast and lunch and only engages in long and intense training throughout the day. When dinner time comes, he eats his one meal of the day. Walker also happens to be a vegetarian, which means that his diet is plant-based. To Walker, it's all about the mindset. He has been eating this way for a long time now, and it makes life easier for him. In fact, he even believes that this type of lifestyle improves his performance. This is one example of how OMAD can also be suitable for you even if you work out or undergo training for sports competitions.

It helps improve your willpower and discipline

Finally, OMAD strengthens your willpower and discipline too. This eating method can be quite challenging, especially for beginners. Sticking with it for the long-run means that you should have a lot of discipline and self-control. Hunger pangs are very powerful, and if you give in to them all the time, you can't really follow this method. On the other hand, if you can master this extreme eating pattern, you will also be honing your willpower and discipline in the process.

As you can see, OMAD comes with a lot of great things too. It makes other IF methods look very easy, whether you are a beginner or not. As long as you learn how to follow it properly —don't worry, there aren't any strict rules, just a few guidelines and suggestions—you can experience all of these benefits and more.

HOW TO FOLLOW THE OMAD METHOD

The OMAD diet is relatively simple. Unlike diets, there aren't any strict rules that you must follow. But just like the other IF methods, OMAD comes with a few guidelines and suggestions that can help make your journey simpler and easier. For instance, it's best to choose a time for when you will have your meal of the day—try to stick with this time consistently. For instance, you can skip breakfast and dinner, and have a big meal at lunch. Personally, I skip breakfast and lunch, then have a big, satisfying dinner. This is the best time for me because I'm not busy, and I get to enjoy my meal without having to rush through it. Of course, the timing would be entirely up to you. Now, here are a few more tips to help you follow this extreme IF method:

1. Ease into the diet

Since this method is quite extreme, it's not recommended to jump right into it right away. For instance, after reading this book, you decide to start following OMAD tomorrow—without a plan and without prior experience. Instead, you may want to think of how you will approach this eating pattern first. Come up with a plan of your own for how to start following OMAD. Give yourself time to adjust to make things much easier for you.

2. Learn how to listen to your body

Learning how to listen to your body is vital if you want to succeed on OMAD or on any other method of IF, for that matter. Even if you eat the healthiest meal each day, there are some bodies that don't do well with fasting for 23 hours each day. If you have such a body, then OMAD might not be the best choice for you. For instance, if you feel stressed all the time, your sleeping patterns are disturbed or you are constantly tired even after you have been following the method for a few months, then you may need to rethink your diet choices. You can modify your IF method based on how it makes your body feel, but you can only do this by learning how to listen to your body and all of its cues.

3. If you are a woman, be more careful

While everyone should practice caution when it comes to OMAD, women should be particularly careful. There have been cases where women experienced suppression of their reproductive hormones because of this extreme method. If you're a woman and you have noticed changes in your monthly cycle after following this eating pattern, have yourself checked. In fact, you may want to have yourself checked first before starting the OMAD method in the first place, especially if you also suffer from any medical condition.

4. Try to watch what you eat

Just because OMAD (and IF in general) focuses more on your timing and not the food that you eat, this doesn't mean that you should eat anything and everything that you want. For instance, having a single meal that consists of chips, fried chicken wings, and a mug of beer isn't the best type of meal to have on OMAD. Such a meal might make you feel full after eating it but it won't sustain you for the rest of the day.

Also, gorging on unhealthy foods every day will put you on a path that's far from the health and wellness goals you expect to achieve through intermittent fasting. As much as possible, it's best to opt for a nutrient-dense, balanced meal each day to ensure that your body is well-nourished. Once in a while, you may indulge in your food cravings. Just pair these with a healthy side dish like a salad to add nutrients to your meal.

5. Make sure your meal counts

Since you will only be having one meal for the day, make sure it counts. This is why I started OMAD by counting calories. Since I was trying to overcome a condition (insulin resistance), I had to make sure that I wasn't depriving myself of the nutrients my body needed to stay healthy. After some time, I didn't have to keep counting calories because I already had a good estimation of the caloric content of my meals. I learned how to prepare and cook my own meals too. This was very helpful. Instead of ordering out, I made sure that all my meals were balanced, healthy, nutrient-dense, satisfying, and they made me feel happy. Cooking my own meals also enabled me to gain a good estimation of the calories that different types of food contain.

6. Be flexible even with the timing

I suggested that you stick with a constant eating time to make it easier for your body to adjust to OMAD. However, this is only a suggestion. This way of eating has worked for me, but if it doesn't work for you, then find your own strategy. For instance, if you want to spread out your large meal over the course of an hour, do that. Or if you have decided to eat your meal at lunchtime but you already feel hungry at breakfast (maybe because you had a lot of activities on the previous day), allow yourself to eat. Don't let the schedule you have set; take control of your life. Being too strict with yourself might make you feel bad, which, in turn, might even push you to give up.

7. Try not to consume a lot of carbs

This is another suggestion that can improve your chances of succeeding in OMAD. Remember that one of the benefits of this eating pattern is autophagy. Also, fasting for long periods of time forces your body into ketosis for it to become an efficient fat-burning machine. However, when you eat a lot of carbs, your body won't achieve ketosis and autophagy until it has burned and used all of the starches and sugars from those carbs completely. Naturally, this will take a longer time if your meal is full of carbs like rice, pasta, bread, and other high-carb food sources. Instead, you may want to opt for healthy fats, proteins, and minimal carbs to make for a more satisfying and filling meal.

8. Know what to eat and what to avoid

In line with the last tip, it would also be a good idea for you to know what are the best foods to eat on OMAD and what are the foods you should limit or avoid. Even though intermittent fasting doesn't involve restricting yourself in terms of the foods you eat, choosing healthy foods will help you reach your health and fitness goals a lot faster. When planning your meals, here are some of the best options to include:

1. **Beverages** like fresh fruit juice, water, seltzer, etc.
2. **Broth**, preferably homemade.
3. **Condiments** like apple cider vinegar, olive oil, salt, pepper, etc.
4. **Dairy** like plain yogurt, cottage cheese, milk, etc.
5. **Fruits** like apples, bananas, mangoes, peaches, kiwis, etc.
6. **Herbs** like parsley, cilantro, basil, etc.
7. **Protein** like eggs, steak, turkey, chicken, fish, etc.
8. **Vegetables** like carrots, leafy greens, cauliflower, celery, garlic, mushrooms, broccoli, zucchini, etc.

You can also include small portions of the following when planning your meals:

1. **Grains** like quinoa, oats, pasta, etc.
2. **Nuts** like almonds, cashews, macadamias, etc.

3. **Seeds** like sunflower seeds, chia seeds, etc.
4. **Starches** like corn, potatoes, beans, etc.

Then there are the foods you may want to avoid, especially when planning your one meal for the day. These are the foods that you may allow yourself to indulge in occasionally, as long as you pair these foods with healthier options. The foods to avoid include:

1. Artificial sweeteners.
2. Cakes, cookies, and other sugary pastries.
3. Chips and other processed snacks.
4. Processed meats.
5. Refined carbs.
6. Sweetened or carbonated beverages with added sugar.
7. Sweets.

As long as you plan your meals well and you make sure that your meals contain all of the nutrients you need to stay healthy, you can eat whatever you want while on OMAD. Also, make sure that your meals make you feel happy and satisfied so that you won't be thinking about food for the rest of the day.

The OMAD method is so simple, but it helps to have a plan for following it. Also, the more you learn about OMAD, the more you can prepare yourself for what's about to come. So, for the last section of this chapter, let me give you a brief introduction of the "dark side" of OMAD to provide you with a clearer look at the whole picture.

THE POTENTIAL RISKS AND DOWNSIDES OF THE OMAD METHOD

We have already established that the OMAD diet is an eating pattern where you would eat one healthy, balanced, and satisfying meal per day within a span of one hour. But for some people, especially the ones who try following this method for the first time, they use their short feeding window to have a massive binge. Obviously, this is not the way to go. Binge eating is never good for your health and when you do it every day, you might experience a decline in your health instead of an improvement.

The OMAD method has a lot of potential benefits, and it's super-easy to follow. However, it's not perfect. As it is, you don't have to worry about the timing of your food because you will only eat one meal each day. This simplicity makes the diet seem too good to be true and for some people, it is. The potential risks and downsides of the OMAD method typically apply to those who don't follow this eating pattern correctly. Here are some examples of situations when OMAD can become troublesome instead of beneficial:

- Some people only eat unhealthy foods for their one meal. If you want the OMAD diet to work for you, it's recommended to have a home-cooked meal that contains vitamins, minerals, and nutrients all in one plate (or bowl).

- Some people don't consume enough protein while focusing only on high-carb foods. This won't work because too many carbs will make you feel hungry after some time. Also, not consuming enough protein might put you at risk for muscle loss.
- Some people who suffer from a condition might need to take medications with their food. Of course, this will be a problem when they only eat one meal a day. In such a case, if you really want to follow OMAD, consult with your doctor first. Find out if there is any way for you to follow this method while still taking your medications.
- Some experts claim that OMAD can potentially slow down your metabolism in the long-run. This may happen if you follow OMAD for a long time as the slowing down of your metabolism is a natural response when you fast for long periods of time. This is why it's important to transition out of OMAD slowly—so that your body can adjust to the changes again.

To avoid the negative side effects of OMAD, your plate should contain the recommended daily amounts of vegetables, fruits, and protein in a single meal. Remember that this meal should be enough to tide you over until the next day. This is just a peek at the things that can go wrong with OMAD. Later, we will discuss these in more detail to help you understand them more. But before that, let me share with you the best tips and strategies for following OMAD (and IF) correctly. That way, you won't have to deal with the negative side effects and potential risks of this extreme method. When you know what to expect and how to overcome issues, there is a higher likelihood that you will succeed in your OMAD journey.

5

PREPARING TO FOLLOW THE OMAD METHOD OF INTERMITTENT FASTING

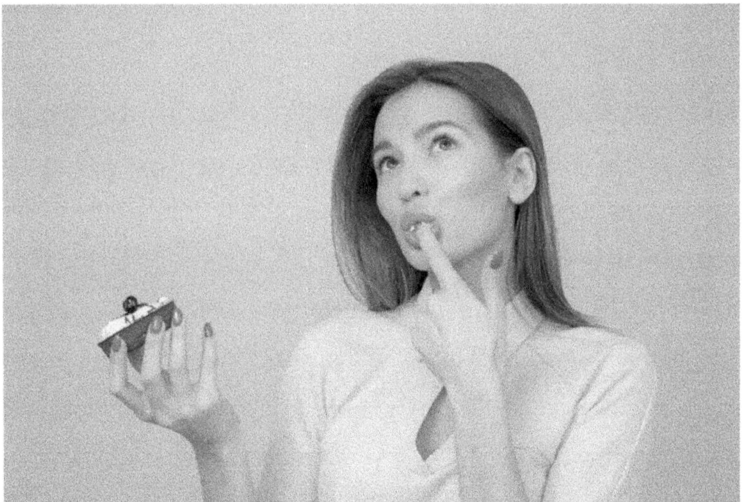

Fig. 7: Getting Ready for OMAD. Unsplash, by Icons8 Team, 2018, https://unsplash.com/photos/NtwdMDylfTw/ Copyright 2018 by Icons8 Team/Unsplash.

Now, it's time to get practical. At this point, you would already have a strong motivation to start following the diet. As soon as you finish reading this book, you can apply everything you have learned to succeed on your OMAD journey. In this chapter, you will be learning everything else that you need to get started. As someone who has been following the OMAD method for some time now, I can tell you that it's totally achievable. I can also tell you that this eating pattern has benefited my life in so many ways. Now, let's prepare you to begin with the OMAD method of intermittent fasting...

START SLOW!

Since the OMAD method is quite extreme, the best way to approach it is by going slow. If it's your first time following intermittent fasting, then you may want to try one of the easier methods first. For instance, you can follow the 16:8 method for a few weeks or months just to help your body adjust and get familiar with fasting. Then you can make modifications to the method you have chosen by gradually increasing the length of your fasting window. To give you a more practical look at how your transition would go, here is an example of the steps you can follow:

- When you feel like you have adjusted to the first method that you are following, start increasing the duration of your fasts. For instance, if you follow the

16:8 method, increase your fasting window to 18 or 20 hours two to three times each week.

- When you feel more comfortable with longer fasts, you can start doing OMAD fasts one to two times a week.
- On Monday, you follow your modified 16:8 fasting method.
- On Tuesday, you follow the OMAD method, wherein you will eat a big meal that contains around 1,200 to 1,300 calories.
- On Wednesday, you have a regular eating day.
- On Thursday, you follow your modified 16:8 fasting method.
- On Friday, you follow the OMAD method, wherein you will eat a big meal that contains around 1,200 to 1,300 calories.
- On Saturday, you have a regular eating day.
- On Sunday, you follow your modified 16:8 fasting method.

This is just an example of how you can transition from your current IF method to OMAD. You can create your own plan and schedule to follow. As you are in the transition phase, don't forget to listen to your body and trust your instincts.

The plan and schedule you create depend on your starting point. For instance, if you have tried fasting in the past (not necessarily intermittent fasting) and you immediately want to try OMAD, then your plan would look different. The key here is to make sure that your health won't get compromised as you start following OMAD. For instance, if you have no fasting experience and you immediately follow the OMAD method every day for a whole week, you might experience a lot of adverse side effects. No matter what your health and fitness goals are, try not to rush through the process. Give yourself—and your body—time to adjust to intermittent fasting. This is true no matter what method you have chosen to follow. As long as you feel comfortable with your process and your body isn't stressed, then you're doing it correctly.

MEAL PLANNING FOR THE OMAD METHOD

Meal planning is a process where you take the time to sit down and plan your meals for a whole week. You can also plan your meals for a specific number of days. But the point is, meal planning is all about... planning your meals! If you already practice meal planning, you can still continue to do so while on OMAD. In fact, meal planning becomes easier when you follow this eating pattern. But if you haven't tried meal planning before, you may want to consider it. Meal planning helps make your life easier, simpler, and healthier.

If you plan to ease into OMAD, then your meal plans for the transition period might be a bit complex. After all, you would have to plan different numbers of meals for different days. For instance, going back to the example I shared in the last schedule, your meal plan for the week would look something like this:

- Monday (16:8): light breakfast, light lunch, and a light snack.
- Tuesday (OMAD): big breakfast.
- Wednesday (regular eating day): breakfast, lunch, snack, dinner.
- Thursday (16:8): light breakfast, light lunch, and a light snack.
- Friday (OMAD): big breakfast.
- Saturday (regular eating day): breakfast, lunch, snack, dinner.
- Sunday (16:8): light breakfast, light lunch, and a light snack.

You may follow this routine for a few weeks before making modifications to move you towards your goal of completely following the OMAD method. Each time you make modifications to your eating pattern, make sure to update your meal plan too. That way, you can shop for, prepare, and cook your meals accordingly. When making your meal plan for OMAD, here are some things for you to keep in mind:

- You aren't required to exclude any foods or food groups. However, it's best to avoid unhealthy foods as much as you can. You may have these indulgences once in a while—just not every day.

- Make sure that the meal you have planned will make you feel full and satisfied. While planning, remember that a lot of recipes are meant for single meal servings. Therefore, you have the option to eat more than a single serving of the dishes you cook or combine the dish with something else to increase the total number of calories.
- Take note of the macronutrient content of your meals. The macronutrients are protein, carbs, and fat. Also, try to make sure that each of your meals contains other essential vitamins, minerals, and nutrients. This will prevent you from developing a nutrient deficiency.
- If you want to be really healthy, focus on vegetables, fruits, high-quality lean proteins (organic, if possible), high-quality dairy products (organic, if possible), and complex carbs. You may also want to add healthy fats to your meals like olive oil and avocados to increase the nutritional value.
- If you don't think that you can eat enough to ensure that you're getting all of the nutrients your body requires to stay healthy, you may consider taking supplements. Before doing this, speak to your doctor first. Your doctor can give you advice on how to plan your meals better and what are the best supplements to take along with your OMAD eating pattern.

Meal planning helps you follow the OMAD method safely and effectively. When you plan your meals, you are also making sure that you're getting enough macro- and micronutrients for each of your meals. That way, you don't have to count your calories when it's time for you to eat. As long as you prepared or cooked the meal, you can also be sure that it is nutritious and filling enough.

If in the past, you had to think about 21 meals a week plus snacks, when you follow OMAD, your meal planning will go down to only seven meals a week. This means that you will save a lot of time and effort with this practical process. Let me share with you another example. This time, I will share a sample meal plan to give you an idea on what a week on OMAD will look like:

- Monday: Mac & cheese, roasted Brussels sprouts, and a turmeric ginger smoothie.
- Tuesday: Mexican-style tortilla soup with lentils, fresh fruit juice, and an apple muffin.
- Wednesday: Chickpea wraps, an avocado salad, and a mango smoothie.
- Thursday: Falafel sandwich with sweet potatoes, overnight oats, and fresh fruit juice.
- Friday: Quinoa power bowl, a piece of fruit, and an almond butter smoothie with blueberries.
- Saturday: Shepherd's pie, dinner rolls, and fruit juice.

- Sunday: Breakfast burritos, a side salad, and an avocado smoothie.

Most of the time, the meals you plan would contain a main meal, a side dish, a beverage, and a dessert if desired. For the rest of the day, continue to hydrate yourself with non-caloric beverages so you don't feel hungry all the time and you won't experience the common side effects of long periods of fasting. In the next section, there are more ideas for you to add to your meal plan. But this time, in the form of recipes.

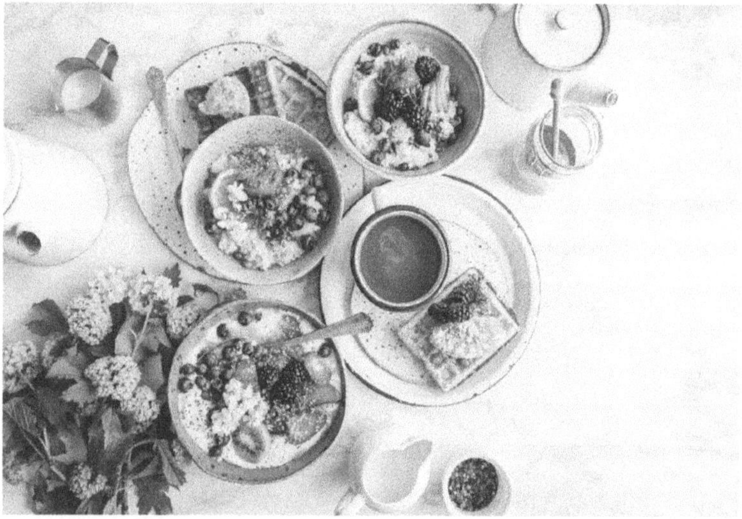

Fig. 8: Recipes. Unsplash, by Brooke Lark, 2017, https://unsplash.com/photos/HlNcigvUi4Q/ Copyright 2017 by Brooke Lark/Unsplash.

7 SUGGESTED RECIPES FOR YOUR OMAD METHOD MEAL PLANNING

Following the OMAD method doesn't have to be challenging. As long as you plan for it, you can ensure that you are getting enough calories each day to avoid compromising your health or developing any nutrient deficiencies. As much as possible, you should consume 1,200 calories on your single meal with the following macronutrient breakdown:

- Carbs: 10 grams
- Fat: 104 grams
- Protein: 105 grams

These are the ideal values, but you can practice flexibility so you won't have to be too strict when planning your meals. Here are a few recipes you can cook as you follow the OMAD method. These recipes are healthy, delicious, filling, and will provide you with the nutrients you need for the day.

Taco Bowl with Steak Strips

This is a low-carb recipe that's simple, healthy, and versatile too. You need only 20 minutes to create the whole dish, and you can even change up the ingredients as you see fit. For the steak strips, you can either cook them for this recipe or you can also use leftovers if you have any. Although this taco bowl requires simple ingredients, it packs a lot of flavors to make you feel satisfied with the single meal for the day.

Time: 20 minutes

Serving Size: 1 taco bowl

Prep Time: 10 minutes

Cook Time: 10 minutes

Nutritional Information:

- *Calories: 702 kcal*
- *Carbs: 8.8 grams*
- *Fat: 56.1 grams*
- *Protein: 34.3 grams*

Ingredients for the steak:

- 1 tsp lime juice (fresh)
- 1 tbsp ghee
- 2 tbsp cilantro (minced)
- ⅓ lb filet steak of your choice
- 1 cup of cauliflower rice (cooked)
- black pepper
- salt

Ingredients for the toppings:

- 1 tbsp sour cream
- ¼ cup of tomato salsa (homemade or store-bought)
- ½ jalapeño (sliced thinly)
- 1 small avocado (peeled, pitted, sliced)
- cilantro (optional, chopped, for garnish)
- 2 lemon wedges (optional, for garnish)

Directions:

- Pat the filet steak dry with a paper towel to remove excess moisture.
- Season the filet steak with salt and black pepper on all sides.
- In a skillet, add the ghee over medium-high heat.
- Add the seasoned filet steak to the skillet and sear on both sides for about 4 to 8 minutes. The cooking time depends on the level of doneness you prefer.
- Transfer the seared filet steak to a cutting board to rest.
- As the filet steak is resting, assemble the taco bowl. Start by adding the cauliflower rice, lime juice, and cilantro to a bowl then mix until well-combined.
- Add all of the topping ingredients and arrange as desired.
- Slice the filet steak into strips and add to the bowl. Garnish with cilantro and lemon wedges if using.
- Serve immediately.

You can also store the taco bowl for one day in the refrigerator. For this meal, you can either increase the quantities of the ingredients to reach the recommended number of calories or you can pair it with a side dish like a salad, a bowl of soup, or a cup of brown rice. A smoothie or a dessert like a peanut butter and banana muffin would be a great addition to this meal too.

Salmon Power Platter

While following the OMAD method, you don't have to create complex dishes for yourself. Here is another simple recipe where all you have to do is prepare all of the ingredients and bring them together in a single platter. This is a wholesome dish that bursts with flavor and nutrients. It also features salmon as the main ingredient, one of the healthiest foods out there. As with the previous recipe, you can also change, add, or replace the ingredients to suit your palate.

Time: 10 minutes

Serving Size: 2 platters (1 platter on OMAD)

Prep Time: 5 minutes

Cook Time: 5 minutes

Nutritional Information:

- *Calories: 537 kcal*
- *Carbs: 4.6 grams*

- *Fat: 39.9 grams*
- *Protein: 36 grams*

Ingredients for the bowl:

- 2 tsp water
- 2 tbsp pumpkin seeds
- 2 tbsp red onion (raw, chopped)
- ½ lb salmon fillet (cooked or smoked, flaked)
- ¼ cup of asparagus (chopped)
- 1 cup of salad greens (rinsed, drained)
- 1 medium avocado (peeled, pitted, sliced)
- 2 hard-boiled eggs (cut in half)

Ingredients for the dressing:

- 1 tsp horseradish
- ½ tbsp capers (finely chopped)
- 1 tbsp apple cider vinegar
- 1 tbsp olive oil
- 1 tbsp parsley (finely chopped)
- 2 tbsp mayonnaise
- black pepper
- salt

Directions:

- Make the dressing by combining all of the ingredients in a bowl. Mix well and set aside.
- After washing the salad greens, drain them on a salad spinner.
- In a microwaveable bowl, add the asparagus and water.
- Place the bowl in the microwave and cook the asparagus on high for about 3 to 6 minutes. The asparagus should have a vibrant green color while retaining the crunchy texture.
- Slice the salmon fillet into strips and place on a platter.
- Add the egg halves, avocado slices, onion, and the cooked asparagus then top with the salad greens.
- Sprinkle the pumpkin seeds all over the salad greens and drizzle with dressing.
- Serve immediately.

This recipe can make up to two servings but if you're on OMAD, you can have both servings for yourself. Then round off this rich and filling meal with a low-carb dessert like a flourless muffin or a low-carb mug cake.

Rainbow Bowl

While following the OMAD method, bowls and platters are the easiest, healthiest, and most filling options for you. This is because they contain several ingredients that you would simply have to bring together to create your meal. Bowl and platter meals are also very flexible allowing you to mix and match according to what you feel like eating for the day. This recipe allows you to "eat the rainbow" as it contains healthy ingredients of different colors.

Time: 25 minutes

Serving Size: 2 bowls (1 bowl on OMAD)

Prep Time: 5 minutes

Cook Time: 20 minutes

Nutritional Information:

- *Calories: 599 kcal*
- *Carbs: 63.6 grams*
- *Fat: 22.1 grams*
- *Protein: 39.5 grams*

Ingredients:

- ½ tsp cooking oil
- ½ tsp garlic powder
- ½ tsp onion powder
- 1 tsp kosher salt
- ½ tbsp cumin (ground)
- ½ tbsp oregano (dried)
- ½ tbsp sweet or hot smoked paprika
- ½ tbsp vegetable oil of your choice

- ¾ tbsp chili powder
- ½ lb ground beef (extra lean)
- ½ cup of corn (canned, drained)
- 1 cup of black beans (canned, rinsed, drained)
- 1 cup of cherry tomatoes (cut into halves)
- 1 cup of sweet potatoes (peeled, cubed)
- 1 small avocado (peeled, pitted, sliced)
- ½ tsp cayenne powder (optional)

Directions:

- Preheat your oven to 400° F.
- In a bowl, combine the garlic powder, salt, onion powder, cumin, oregano, paprika, and chili powder. Add cayenne pepper, if using, and mix everything together until well-combined.
- In a baking sheet, add the sweet potato cubes.
- Drizzle with vegetable oil and sprinkle half of the seasoning mixture.
- Toss the sweet potato cubes lightly until all pieces are evenly coated.
- Place the baking sheet in the oven and bake the sweet potato cubes for about 15 to 20 minutes until completely cooked through and tender.
- In the meantime, add cooking oil to a pan over medium heat.
- Once the oil is hot, add the ground beef and cook for

about 5 to 7 minutes. The ground beef must be completely cooked through. If excess oils are released from the ground beef, drain carefully. Just leave around 1 tablespoon of fat.

- Add the black beans to the pan along with the rest of the seasoning mixture.
- Toss the ingredients together until the ground beef and black beans are fully coated with oil and seasonings.
- Continue cooking until the beans are completely heated through. Keep tossing so that the ingredients won't stick to the pan.
- Add all of the ingredients in a bowl (the cooked and raw ingredients). Arrange as desired and serve immediately.

You can have both servings to yourself, and these would provide you with enough calories for the day. But you can also add more toppings like crumbled feta, jalapeños, sour cream, or green onion to make this bowl more flavorful. Then enjoy it with a refreshing glass of lemonade for a hearty, healthy meal.

Vegan Burritos

Burritos are very filling, especially when you use the right ingredients. This recipe offers a vegan twist to burritos, but you can also add some protein to it like steak slices, ground beef or shredded chicken. Doing this will add more calories to the dish, thus, bringing you closer to your daily caloric intake target. This is another easy recipe that comes together in just half an hour.

Time: 30 minutes

Serving Size: 2 burritos

Prep Time: 15 minutes

Cook Time: 15 minutes

Nutritional Information:

- *Calories: 713 kcal*
- *Carbs: 131 grams*
- *Fat: 14 grams*
- *Protein: 19 grams*

Ingredients for the filling:

- ¼ tsp chili powder
- ¼ tsp cumin
- ¼ tsp garlic powder
- 1 tbsp lime juice (fresh)
- 2 tbsp butter
- ¼ cup of cilantro (fresh, chopped)
- ¾ cup of rice (cooked)
- 1 cup of black beans (cooked with a pinch of salt, drained)

- 1 small red onion (sliced)
- 2 medium red potatoes (washed, peeled, cubed)
- black pepper
- sea salt

Ingredients for the slaw:

- 2 tbsp lime juice (fresh)
- 1 cup of purple cabbage (thinly sliced)
- ¼ medium avocado
- 1 jalapeño (seeds removed, sliced)
- black pepper
- sea salt

Ingredients for serving:

- ¼ cup of salsa (homemade or store-bought)
- ½ medium avocado (sliced)
- 2 large flour tortillas of your choice)
- hot sauce of your choice (optional)

Directions:

- In a skillet, add the butter over medium heat and swirl around to coat the whole surface.
- Add the potato cubes on one side of the skillet and the

chopped onion on the other. Sprinkle with sea salt and black pepper.

- Cover the skillet and allow the vegetables to cook for about 4 to 5 minutes.
- Remove the cover, toss or flip the vegetables over, replace the cover, and continue cooking for about 4 to 5 minutes until golden brown.
- Remove the skillet from the heat then set aside.
- In a saucepan, add the beans over medium heat. Sprinkle with chili powder, garlic powder, and cumin.
- Mix the beans to coat them with the seasonings.
- When the beans release water and start bubbling, bring the heat down to low to keep the beans warm.
- In a bowl, add the avocado and mash. Add the lime juice and mix well.
- Add the jalapeño and cabbage then toss together to combine.
- Season with sea salt and black pepper, toss lightly, then set aside.
- Prepare the cooked rice by adding cilantro and lime juice. Use a fork to toss lightly.
- Warm the flour tortillas in the microwave for about 30 seconds. This will soften them too.
- Start assembling the tortillas. Add half of the rice to each tortilla.
- Continue adding the rest of the filling ingredients to the tortillas in any order.

- Top each of the tortillas with the avocado slaw, avocado slices, salsa, and hot sauce, if using.
- Wrap the burritos carefully and serve immediately.

If you have any leftover toppings, you can serve them on the side. You can have both burritos in one sitting but it might be too filling for you. Instead, you can store one of the burritos in the refrigerator and pair the other one with a filling side dish like a baked chicken breast or a pan-fried salmon fillet. You can also round off your meal with a decadent dessert like crème brulée or a slice of blueberry cheesecake.

Full-English Breakfast Plate

Here's a filling platter for you to enjoy at any time of the day. It's healthy, colorful, scrumptious, and oh-so-easy to bring together. Again, you can change some of the ingredients according to your preference. Just make sure that the ingredients you replace will help you reach your caloric intake target while adding variety to your meal. This tip applies to the other recipes too.

Time: 15 minutes

Serving Size: 1 plate

Prep Time: 5 minutes

Cook Time: 10 minutes

Nutritional Information:

- *Calories: 658 kcal*
- *Carbs: 7 grams*
- *Fat: 55 grams*
- *Protein: 29.6 grams*

Ingredients:

- 1 tbsp duck fat or ghee
- ½ cup of spinach (fresh, rinsed, drained)
- 1 small avocado (peeled, pitted, sliced)
- 2 large eggs
- 2 to 3 slices of bacon
- 5 to 6 brown mushrooms
- 5 to 6 cherry tomatoes (still on the vine)
- black pepper
- salt
- chili pepper flakes (optional)
- 2 Italian sausages (optional, for added protein)

Directions:

- In a skillet, add the duck fat over medium-high heat.
- Add the mushrooms with their top side-down.
- Season with salt and black pepper then cook for about 5 minutes.

- Flip the mushrooms over and continue cooking for about 2 minutes until tender.
- Take the cooked mushrooms out of the skillet and set aside.
- In a pan, fry the bacon over medium heat until your desired level of doneness.
- Once cooked, place on a paper towel to drain excess oils.
- In the same pan, fry the eggs according to your preference.
- Once cooked, transfer to your serving plate.
- Turn up the heat to high, add the vine of cherry tomatoes, and cook for about 1 minute. If you want to serve the tomatoes raw, you can skip this step.
- If you want to add Italian sausages to your platter, cook them on the same pan too.
- Add all of the ingredients (cooked and raw) to the serving platter along with the eggs. Arrange them as desired.
- Top with avocado slices and serve immediately.

This amazing dish bursts with different flavors and textures. On its own, it's quite filling already. But you can also pair it with a thick and creamy bowl of roasted squash soup or a decadent dessert like apple pie a la mode.

Warm and Rich Coconut Curry

This recipe is simple, packed with veggies, and full of flavors. It's a definite crowd-pleaser that's gluten-free and vegan too. Although this is one of the lighter options I will share with you, it's great on OMAD because you can pair it with different side dishes to create a hearty, healthy meal for the day.

Time: 30 minutes

Serving Size: 2 bowls (1 bowl for OMAD)

Prep Time: 5 minutes

Cook Time: 25 minutes

Nutritional Information:

- *Calories: 434 kcal*
- *Carbs: 41 grams*
- *Fat: 25.8 grams*
- *Protein: 10.2 grams*

Ingredients:

- ½ tbsp curry powder
- ½ tbsp ginger (fresh, grated)
- ½ tbsp olive oil
- ⅛ cup of snow peas (sliced in half)
- ⅛ cup of tomatoes (diced)
- ¼ cup of broccoli florets (diced)

- ¼ cup of carrots (diced)
- ½ cup of vegetable broth (homemade or store-bought)
- 1 cup of coconut quinoa (cooked using 1 ¾ cup of coconut milk)
- 1 ¾ cup of coconut milk
- 1 small onion (diced)
- 2 cloves of garlic (minced)
- black pepper
- sea salt
- ½ tsp cayenne powder (optional, for cooking)
- ½ tsp red pepper flakes (optional, for serving)
- 2 lemon wedges (optional, for serving)

Directions:

- Start by cooking the coconut quinoa.
- In a pot, add the coconut oil over medium heat.
- Add the garlic, onion, carrots, broccoli florets, ginger, sea salt, and black pepper then stir to combine.
- Cook the vegetables for about 5 minutes until softened. Stir frequently so the vegetables don't stick to the bottom of the pot.
- Add the coconut milk, vegetable broth, curry powder, salt, black pepper, and cayenne powder if using.
- Mix the ingredients together and bring to a boil.
- Once boiling, lower the heat slightly, and simmer for about 10 to 15 minutes. While cooking, taste the

mixture and add more seasonings according to your preference.

- In the last 5 minutes of cooking, add the tomatoes and snow peas.
- Pour the curry into a bowl and garnish with lemon wedges and red pepper, if using.
- Serve immediately with coconut quinoa.

Note: To cook the coconut quinoa, add ½ tablespoon of cooking oil to a saucepan over medium heat. Add 1 cup of quinoa and cook for about 5 minutes until golden. Stir often so it doesn't burn. Add 1½ cups of water, 1 ¾ cups of coconut milk, and a pinch of salt then mix well. Bring the mixture to a boil and turn the heat down to low. Cover the saucepan and allow to simmer for about 20 to 25 minutes until all of the liquid has evaporated and the quinoa is cooked. Use a fork to fluff and set aside while you prepare the curry dish.

If you will eat both servings, then you can round off your meal with a decadent dessert like a chocolate lava cake. But if you will only have one bowl of this curry with half of the coconut quinoa, then you can complete your meal with some kind of protein like grilled chicken or a baked fillet of fish.

Pan-Fried Pork Chop with Hollandaise Sauce and Asparagus

This last dish would be perfect for an easy and quick weeknight dinner. It's the perfect combination of sweet asparagus, tender pork chops, and a lovely hollandaise sauce that ties all the flavors together. You can even use the sauce for other dishes once you've learned how to make it.

Time: 35 minutes

Serving Size: 1 serving

Prep Time: 10 minutes

Cook Time: 25 minutes

Nutritional Information:

- *Calories: 690 kcal*
- *Carbs: 2.8 grams*
- *Fat: 58.8 grams*
- *Protein: 36 grams*

Ingredients:

- 1 tbsp ghee
- 1 tbsp lemon juice (fresh)
- ½ cup of butter (melted)
- ¾ cup of asparagus spears
- 1 pork loin chop (bone-in)
- 3 large eggs (yolks only)
- salt
- black pepper

Directions:

- Start by preparing the hollandaise sauce first. In a jar with a wide mouth, add the butter. The mouth of the jar should be wide enough so that you can fit a hand blender into it. If you don't have such a jar, make the sauce in a microwaveable bowl first then transfer into a jar.
- Add the lemon juice and egg yolks in the butter, then blend with a hand blender.
- As you're blending, lift the hand blender slowly. Taste the sauce and add salt and black pepper according to your preference. Set the sauce aside.
- Add the ghee in a pan over medium-high heat.
- Add the pork chop to the pan and cook one side for about 6 minutes.
- Flip the pork chop over and continue cooking the other side for another 6 minutes.
- Take the pork chop out of the pan and allow it to rest for about 5 minutes.
- In a pot, add water (enough to submerge the asparagus spears), and bring to a boil.
- Once boiling, add the asparagus spears and blanch for about 5 minutes.
- Take the asparagus spears out of the water. Drain well.
- On a plate, add the pork chop and the asparagus spears on the side.

- Drizzle with the homemade hollandaise sauce and serve.

Since this recipe calls for the use of raw eggs, you may opt for pasteurized eggs to be on the safer side. Store the rest of the sauce in the refrigerator for up to 4 days with an airtight lid. Warm it a bit before use. You can make this meal more filling by having a cup of rice with it or a thick, hearty soup. If not, you can also end the meal with an indulgent dessert like a soufflé.

OTHER ESSENTIAL TIPS

Although intermittent fasting, specifically the OMAD method isn't a diet, it still involves making changes in your eating habits. I have already shared with you some of the most practical guidelines for following this eating pattern. Now, let us go through a few essential tips to increase your chances of following this extreme IF method:

1. Make sure that you are properly hydrated throughout the day

At one time each day, you will enjoy your full, healthy meal. Before and after that meal, you can still consume non-caloric beverages to ensure that you don't get dehydrated. Some examples of non-caloric beverages are plain coffee, tea, and, of course, water. Maintaining proper hydration is essential, especially if you want to lose weight on OMAD. If you feel hungry at any point before or after your meal, drinking the recommended beverages can help you control your hunger pangs and cravings. The longer you follow OMAD, the more you will notice that your cravings and hunger pangs are diminishing too.

Here's a practical tip for you in terms of hydration—drinking a glass of sparkling water with fresh lemon or lime juice in the morning can help boost your electrolyte levels. OMAD tends to throw off your electrolyte levels, thus, it is important to replenish your electrolytes to ensure your health. You can also add magnesium powder or salt to a glass of water to achieve the same effect. Also, it's more effective to have this glass of water in the morning.

2. Learn how to cook your meals so that you can enjoy a wide variety of dishes

One of the best benefits of meal planning is that it allows you to diversify your diet to keep it interesting. You might think that OMAD will trigger food cravings, and if you eat the same thing each day, you will probably get bored with this eating pattern. On the other hand, if you vary your foods each day, you can make this extreme IF method more interesting, fulfilling, and motivating.

Aside from meal planning, cooking your own meals also allows you to change things up. Cooking can be a very relaxing hobby. When you gain confidence in your cooking skills, you can start looking for more exotic recipes to excite your taste buds. Basically, indulging in a wide variety of foods makes it easier to follow OMAD or any other intermittent fasting method.

3. Eat foods from different food groups

Since you will only be eating once a day, make sure that your plate is filled with foods from different food groups. For instance, if you love eating steaks, it's not the best idea to simply eat one big steak a day and nothing else. Instead, you can have different kinds of steaks that you would pair with a side of buttered vegetables, a light salad, mashed potatoes, or a bowl of soup. This variety makes it easier for you to consume all of the nutrients your body needs each day.

Speaking of steaks, while following OMAD, your plate should always contain a source of protein. Biologically speaking, protein is the most important nutrient you should have. Aside from being good for your health, protein is also filling. Therefore, a meal with a good protein source can help tide you over until the next day when it's time for you to eat your next meal.

4. Stay productive while following the OMAD method

One of the benefits of the OMAD method is better concentration and focus. As these improve, so will your productivity. Take advantage of this benefit by trying to stay productive throughout the day. Staying productive offers two advantages. First, you will have the chance to do everything you need to accomplish for the day. For instance, if you are swamped at work, you will have the time (along with focus and concentration) to accomplish everything without having to think about when or what you will eat during your break time.

The second benefit of staying productive is it can help distract you from the hunger you feel. This is especially helpful at the beginning of your OMAD journey when you are likely to feel hunger or cravings. If you're distracted or busy with your tasks at home or at work, you won't be thinking about your hunger or the fact that your next meal is still hours away.

5. Learn how to relax and make sure that you're always getting enough sleep

At some point, you might feel like OMAD is taking a toll on your health. Since you will be restricting your calories through your eating pattern, you have to make sure that all the other aspects of your life are taken care of too. Relaxation can help make things a lot easier for you. If you feel stressed because you think that you cannot make it to your next meal, try performing relaxation techniques like taking a long soak in the bathtub with a cup of tea or meditation, for example. These activities will help you overcome such feelings. Of course, if they don't go away and you can't focus on anything else, you can give in and allow yourself to eat a light snack. You may have to do this a few times in the beginning.

Getting enough sleep is also essential to your health. Think about it: if you follow an extreme eating pattern like OMAD and you get only three or four hours of sleep each night, you might end up getting ill. You will experience fatigue, dizziness, and other common side effects. But if you make sure that you get enough sleep each night, you are also giving your body a chance to repair and refresh itself for the next day.

6. Engage in light exercises

If you work out regularly, you don't have to stop while following the OMAD diet. However, you may want to decrease the intensity of your workouts, especially when you're starting out. But if you're used to high-intensity workouts, make sure to have your one meal of the day after your workout session. This ensures that you replenish the resources you lost while working out.

If you plan to ease into the OMAD method, then it's recommended to work out on days when you are not scheduled to follow OMAD. For instance, in the example I shared in the meal planning section, the OMAD days are on Tuesday and Friday. This means that you can work out on Monday, Wednesday, Thursday, Saturday, and Sunday. It's all about planning your schedule and your exercise activities to make sure that neither your health nor your workout routine gets compromised.

7. Consider using an app to help you out

These days, there are apps for virtually anything—even for following OMAD. One example of such an app is Cronometer. This app helps you make sure that you are always meeting your recommended daily requirements as you follow the OMAD method. With this app, you can keep track of your calories, log the meals you eat, add notes, create custom foods, and more. If you think that you need all the help you can get to succeed on this diet, then apps like Cronometer can help you out.

8. Change things up once in a while

Finally, it would be more beneficial for you to change your eating pattern once in a while. Although OMAD is highly effective and easy to follow, changing up your method once in a while prevents metabolic adaptation. The changes will keep your body guessing so that you don't have to worry about your metabolism slowing down because it's too used to being "starved." Changing your eating pattern once in a while is the smarter and more sustainable way to approach OMAD.

As you can see, all of these tips are practical, easy, and effective. Although you don't have to follow these tips (and the ones I shared earlier), keeping them in mind while you follow OMAD will help improve your chances of experiencing benefits from it. Of course, you should also know if this eating pattern is no longer working for you.

WHEN TO STOP

The OMAD diet isn't for everyone—I cannot stress this enough. Although it works well for me and for every other proponent of the OMAD method, it might not work for you. Although you might feel disappointed about this, you should still know when to stop. For one, if OMAD is making you sick, stop. If you are suffering from a medical condition and it is getting worse because of OMAD, stop. If you consult with your doctor and they tell you that this eating pattern isn't suitable for you, listen to your doctor. Although OMAD can potentially change your life for the better, if it isn't happening for you, know when to stop. Your health and safety should always be your priority. If OMAD isn't right for you, give the other methods a try.

This is why you should learn how to listen to your body—so that you can determine whether you can continue with OMAD or you should discontinue it. This method might not be alright for you and that's okay. Intermittent fasting can be done in different ways. Maybe another method would work better for you. Or maybe you just need more time for your body to adjust. After following a different method for some time, then you may consider giving OMAD a try again. It's also important for you to be aware of the potential risks and side effects of the OMAD method. This awareness will help you make better choices as you follow the eating pattern or if you choose to stop.

6

THE POTENTIAL RISKS AND SIDE EFFECTS OF THE OMAD METHOD

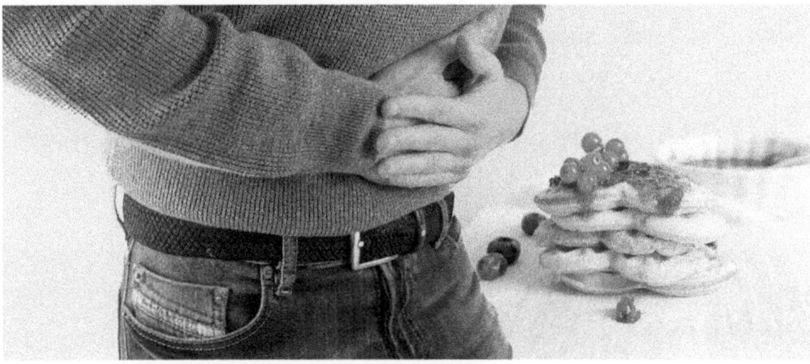

Fig. 9: Hunger. Pixabay, by mohamed Hassan, 2018, https://pixabay.com/photos/stomach-health-diet-dessert-eating-3532098/ Copyright 2018 by mohamed Hassan/Unsplash.

At this point, you have almost everything you need to start following the OMAD method. But I want to share with you all of the essential aspects of this eating pattern for you to make an informed decision on whether to follow it or not.

This means that I will also be sharing with you the "other side of the coin."

While there might be a lot of resources about OMAD online, most of them only have a single focus. Some only focus on the good sides while some only focus on the bad sides. If you only look at the good side of OMAD, you might start following the eating pattern without knowing what to expect or what to avoid. On the other hand, if you only focus on the bad side of OMAD, then you probably won't even bother learning more. This means that you would have wasted an opportunity to make a positive change in your life.

Now that I have shared with you all of the good things to expect from the OMAD method, it's time to learn the potential risks and side effects. Then you can decide whether this method is right for you or if you want to try other methods first.

THE RISKS OF OMAD AND OTHER INTERMITTENT FASTING METHODS

Just like any other extreme diet or eating plan, OMAD comes with its own set of risks. Beneficial as it is, it can also pose dangers to your health, which is why I keep reminding you that this eating method isn't for everyone. But if you are aware of these risks, you might have a better chance of avoiding them. Also, knowing the potential risks of OMAD allows you to recognize them as soon as they start happening to you. As you consider following OMAD or while you are following this eating pattern, look out for these risks:

1. You will experience hunger pangs like never before

This is one of the most common risks of the OMAD method. Eating once a day is very different from eating three times a day, plus having one or two snacks in between. Naturally, when you start fasting, then you will experience frequent hunger pangs. These, in turn, can lead to cravings. Once you give in to your cravings, then you might develop a problematic relationship with food. Even if you can get through your hunger pangs, you might end up binge eating on every meal. Even if you only have one meal a day, this can be very troublesome for you if you binge every day.

If you want to overcome this issue or avoid this risk, expect to experience hunger. Since you will be skipping meals and only eating a single meal each day, the natural response of your body is to feel hungry. As much as possible, try to resist the urge to eat. You can distract yourself with different activities, drink some kind of non-caloric beverage or do anything else that will help take your mind off your hunger. However, if you feel like you cannot control your hunger anymore and it's starting to take a toll on you, then you can eat something light and healthy to tide you over. Remember—you should never compromise your health and well-being.

If you discover that this eating pattern is causing you to binge eat every day, then you may want to re-think your decision to follow the OMAD method. Maybe give yourself more time to adjust to fasting by following a different method first. After your body has adjusted to an easier IF method, then you can try following OMAD again. Hopefully, this time, you can handle your hunger and cravings better.

2. You could get dehydrated if you don't drink enough water

One of the tips I have shared with you in the previous chapters is to keep drinking water and other non-caloric beverages throughout your fasting window. This is very important so that you don't end up getting dehydrated while fasting. This is especially important if you lead an active lifestyle or you are doing a lot of things during your fasting window. Dehydration is very serious, so you must avoid this at all costs. Fortunately, this risk is easier to avoid. All you have to do is be conscious of your liquid intake. No matter how busy you are, make sure that you're drinking enough to keep you hydrated throughout the day.

3. You may experience fatigue, tiredness, and difficulty concentrating

These risks are quite common, especially at the beginning. Since you will be reducing your caloric intake significantly, you would be at risk of experiencing these symptoms. To avoid any issues, easing into the OMAD method is key. Then you can schedule this method on days when you don't have a lot of work or physical activity to do. During your fasting window, you can perform relaxing activities to take your mind off your hunger while avoiding fatigue, tiredness, and difficulty concentrating.

4. You could develop nutritional deficiencies

This is one of the more dangerous risks of the OMAD method. Again, it can come from the caloric restriction that you would be imposing on yourself because you would only be eating one meal each day. You can avoid this risk by making sure that each meal you consume contains a healthy balance of vegetables, fruits, proteins, healthy fats, and complex carbohydrates. Even though you are technically allowed to eat anything you want while on OMAD, it's still recommended to focus on healthy, whole foods to ensure that you won't develop nutrient deficiencies.

Go to your doctor regularly to have your nutrient levels checked. If you find out that you are lacking in specific nutrients, increase your intake of foods that contain those nutrients. Otherwise, you may consider taking supplements after asking your doctor if this is the right step to take.

5. You may experience appetite deregulation

When you shift to OMAD or any other IF method, your appetite changes. In the past, your body would already have an idea of when it's time to eat because you have been following the same eating pattern every day. As you transition into intermittent fasting, you may notice that your appetite isn't the same as it was in the past. While this might not be considered much of a risk to some people, appetite deregulation may also have an effect on your mood.

The reason for this is that the part of the brain that regulates the appetite is the same part of the brain that regulates mood. When nutrient consumption is affected, and appetite deregulation happens, you might experience changes in your mood too. One of the most common changes is irritability—and you might experience this while you are fasting. For this risk, the best thing you can do is try to eat healthily. That way, your body won't suffer because of a lack of nutrients. You can also try relaxation techniques to help make you feel better while you are fasting.

6. Your metabolism might slow down

Finally, if you follow OMAD long term, your metabolism might start slowing down. It won't work efficiently simply because it doesn't have to. Then when you shift back to a normal diet, you might gain a lot of weight. This is why it's recommended to change your method once in a while. That way, your body won't get used to OMAD so much that the slowing down becomes a permanent effect.

These are the most common risks of the OMAD diet. I have also shared some tips on how to avoid them. As long as you are aware of the changes happening to your body and you always listen to your body, there is a good chance that you can avoid these risks. However, if you think that these risks are too much for you to handle, then you may want to come up with your own plan for how to deal with and overcome them if you still want to follow the OMAD method.

SIGNS THAT THE OMAD METHOD ISN'T FOR YOU

The potential risks of the OMAD method aren't the only things to be aware of when you start following it. A lot of us have thrived while following this method but for some people, they realize at some point that OMAD isn't right for them. In such a case, you can either change your approach to the eating pattern or find another method to follow. Either way, if you experience the following signs, it might mean that OMAD isn't the best lifestyle choice for you. Just like being aware of the risks so that you can recognize them when they happen, it's important to look out for these signs that you and OMAD aren't a good fit:

1. If you start becoming obsessed with food

As I had been successful in my own OMAD journey, I can tell you that over time, it gets easier. In the beginning, I was always thinking about my next meal: when I would have it, what I would eat, and how many more hours I would have to wait before I can enjoy another big meal. As the weeks went by, I learned how to distract myself by doing more productive things. I also made sure to hydrate myself throughout the day, so I wouldn't have to think about the hunger I was feeling. Without even realizing it, I had already stopped focusing on my one meal of the day. It became part of my routine.

But when you start becoming obsessed with food, that's a different story. For some people, once they finish their one meal of the day, they feel satisfied. But after a while, their thoughts go back to the food they ate. Then they start feeling overly concerned about what their next meal will be and when they can eat again. If you experience this, it can be an indicator that the OMAD method isn't for you. The main problem with developing an obsession with food is that it may lead to an eating disorder. So if you can't stop thinking about food and it's starting to take over your life, you may have to rethink your choice.

2. If you start feeling guilty about eating

Eating is a natural thing. In fact, it's a necessity. So when you eat your one meal of the day, you should enjoy and relish the experience. After all, this meal is meant to nourish your body and keep you healthy. Since you will only be eating one meal a day, then the meal would be substantially bigger than what you're used to. However, if you feel guilty about consuming so much—even when you know that this is the only meal you will have for the day—then the OMAD method becomes a negative experience for you.

Feelings of guilt or even self-shaming are never good for your well-being. As you transition into OMAD, learn how to be kind to yourself. If you can't stick with the eating pattern rigidly, forgive yourself. Don't berate yourself for giving in to your hunger and eating a light snack. But if the negative feelings don't go away no matter how much you try to convince yourself to be kinder, then this might be another indication that OMAD isn't right for you.

3. When you feel excessive levels of stress

Intermittent fasting tends to increase your cortisol levels. Since OMAD is an extreme method of IF, this means that you might experience high levels of this hormone, which, in turn, makes you feel excessive levels of stress. While OMAD potentially offers a lot of health benefits, if it makes you too stressed to function normally, then this eating pattern might not be the best choice for you to make right now. Before giving up, give relaxation techniques a try. If they work, good for you! You can keep going. But if they don't, then you may have to try other methods of fasting intermittently.

4. When you frequently feel "hangry"

Have you ever felt hangry before? This occurs when you feel so hungry that virtually anything can set you off. A lot of people who start diets or embark on new eating patterns may experience feeling hangry. This is normal. But, again, if you are on OMAD and you notice that you're always hangry, it's time to make a change. Think about it: if you follow OMAD every day, this means that you will feel hangry every day too. Do you really want this feeling to be part of your life? If not, then you may want to find a different method—one that doesn't make you feel hangry all the time.

5. When you feel like "something is off"

If you learn how to listen to your body, you will know what it feels like to be healthy, and you will also know if something's wrong. As you follow OMAD, it's important to listen to your body's cues by increasing your awareness. If you feel like your health is declining and you aren't getting all the nutrients you need to stay healthy, it's time to make a change. You may try modifying your one meal of the day first. Opt for healthier and more diverse foods. You may even increase your caloric intake a bit. But if these changes don't improve the way you feel, if you still feel like something's off, then OMAD might not be for you.

6. When you cannot sleep well

For some people, OMAD might be causing such big changes in their bodies that they start experiencing sleep disturbances like insomnia. Such effects are a huge no-no since sleep is critical to your health. No matter what diet or eating pattern you are following, getting enough sleep every night should be part of the equation. But if fasting is causing issues with your sleeping patterns, then maybe you should try something else.

If you experience any of these signs, don't give up right away. Remember that OMAD is a flexible method just like all the other IF methods available. Consider your approach first and try making a few changes. If the changes you make solve your issue, then you can continue following OMAD. But if you still experience these issues no matter how many times you have tweaked your approach to the OMAD method, then you can make the choice to start following a different IF method.

In such a case, you must already have an exit strategy. Although you want to succeed on OMAD, having a plan to transition out of this method is a wise thing. Even if you succeed, you might choose to go back to your old eating habits after some time. When you reach this point, then you would need your exit strategy too. This will make it easier for you to go back to your old eating patterns without worrying that all of the benefits will go away. It's all about learning how to use your diet and eating patterns to your advantage so that you can achieve your long-term health goals.

WHO SHOULDN'T FOLLOW INTERMITTENT FASTING?

In general, intermittent fasting isn't a good fit for everyone. Whether you choose OMAD or any other method of intermittent fasting, you will be making a commitment to changing your eating pattern in a big way. If you decide to skip meals once in a while just because you're not hungry, you can't really say that you're following IF. While spontaneous meal skipping can be a way for you to start on IF, committing to any of the IF methods is a different thing.

Intermittent fasting offers a number of benefits. However, there are certain groups of people who shouldn't be following this eating pattern. In this last section, we will be going through the different groups of people who should follow IF, those who should consider it very carefully, and those who shouldn't even attempt to follow the diet. Try to see which group you fall under so that you can decide whether it's time for you to follow IF or if you need to make any other preparations before you start, especially if you're planning to follow OMAD.

People who can follow intermittent fasting freely

Generally, there are people who have a higher likelihood of succeeding in IF. Although I didn't technically fall into any of these categories, I had the drive and commitment to follow this trendy eating pattern. I also made sure that I learned everything I can about IF before following it. You can follow IF freely if you:

- Have tried dieting before.
- Have experience monitoring your caloric intake.
- Are healthy and you have a regular workout routine.
- Have a job that allows you to make changes in your eating patterns even if it means having to undergo the potential effects of the transition period.

- Are single or you live alone.
- Don't have any children.
- Have a partner who follows IF or if your partner is open and supportive of your dietary decisions.
- You're a man.

If you fall into any of these categories, then starting on IF might be easier for you. However, even if you're at the peak of health, it's still recommended to talk to your doctor first before you start on IF. You can even have a blood test to check if you have any issues that you don't know about. These steps can give you more confidence in yourself to start following intermittent fasting.

People who should consider this lifestyle change carefully first

If you don't fall into any of the previous categories, then you may want to proceed with caution when it comes to intermittent fasting. If you belong to the following categories, think about this change in lifestyle first and come up with a plan before you start:

- Your job requires you to be at your highest performance all the time. This might make it difficult for you to transition into OMAD.
- You are married, you have children or you live with other people in your home. It might be challenging to

stick with fasting when the rest of your family eat all throughout the day.

- You are an athlete, you compete in sports or you have a strict training regimen. In such a case, you may want to check with your coach or doctor first to ensure that your performance won't get compromised.
- You're a woman. Remember that women should be more cautious when approaching IF.

If you fall into any of these categories, this doesn't mean that you shouldn't follow intermittent fasting. It just means that you should be more careful if you decide to start fasting intermittently. Check with your doctor, educate yourself, and come up with a plan for IF to increase your chances of success.

PEOPLE WHO SHOULDN'T FOLLOW INTERMITTENT FASTING

Finally, there are certain groups of people who shouldn't try intermittent fasting at all. If you fall into any of these categories, try to think of other ways to improve your health. Otherwise, try to improve or change your situation first before you even consider going on IF. It's not recommended for you to follow intermittent fasting if:

You're pregnant or breastfeeding

If you're pregnant or breastfeeding, you need extra energy, thus, you shouldn't be fasting. If you're pregnant, fasting might have adverse effects on the developing fetus in your womb. If you're breastfeeding, you might not have enough nutrients to produce milk for your baby. So it's best to wait until your little one is old enough before you should consider following IF.

You're chronically stressed

Remember that IF can cause you to feel stressed. If you already suffer from chronic stress, going on IF might exacerbate your condition. Learn how to manage your stress better first before you try fasting intermittently.

You have never tried dieting, fasting or exercising before

Although IF can help you lose weight, it's not a good idea for you to follow this eating pattern if you have never tried following a diet, you never exercise or you have never experienced fasting before. Try to prepare your body for intermittent fasting first by developing a workout routine. Then you can also try skipping meals once in a while so you can experience what it feels like to fast. Whatever you do, don't try to jump into IF right away as it might do more harm to your health than good.

You have a history of or you are currently suffering from an eating disorder

Intermittent fasting can make you feel like you're struggling with food. This, in turn, might re-awaken your bad relationship with food, thus, causing more problems for you. Even if you had successfully overcome an eating disorder, you might be at risk for it recurring if you follow intermittent fasting.

You suffer from type 1 diabetes

Although IF can be beneficial for people who suffer from type 2 diabetes, it might not be the best option for those who suffer from type 1 diabetes. This is mainly because you won't be eating meals regularly. If you suffer from this condition and you really want to follow IF, even the simplest method, consult with your doctor and the rest of your health care team first.

OTHER PEOPLE WHO SHOULDN'T FOLLOW IF

- Women trying to conceive.
- Children and teenagers.
- People who suffer from kidney problems.
- People who suffer from adrenal problems.
- People who are underweight.
- People who are taking medications that require regular consumption of meals.
- People who already have sleeping disturbances.

If you fall under any of these categories, then you may want to consider another dietary approach to improve your health. Of course, if you can improve your current situation then you may consider IF sometime in the future. It's also not recommended to start fasting intermittently if this eating pattern doesn't fit into your lifestyle or routine. Now that you know pretty much everything about IF, specifically about the OMAD method, you should already have a good idea of whether this is the right path for you to take or not.

One last thing I would like to say in favor of intermittent fasting is the benefit of customization. Unlike diets, intermittent fasting allows you to customize the method you choose according to your needs. This is one of the most important reasons why so many people succeed on this diet. If you really want to give it a try, don't forget this aspect of the diet. Keep making changes while keeping the basic concept of the method you have chosen until you find the perfect way for you to live comfortably while following intermittent fasting.

CONCLUSION: YOUR INTERMITTENT FASTING JOURNEY

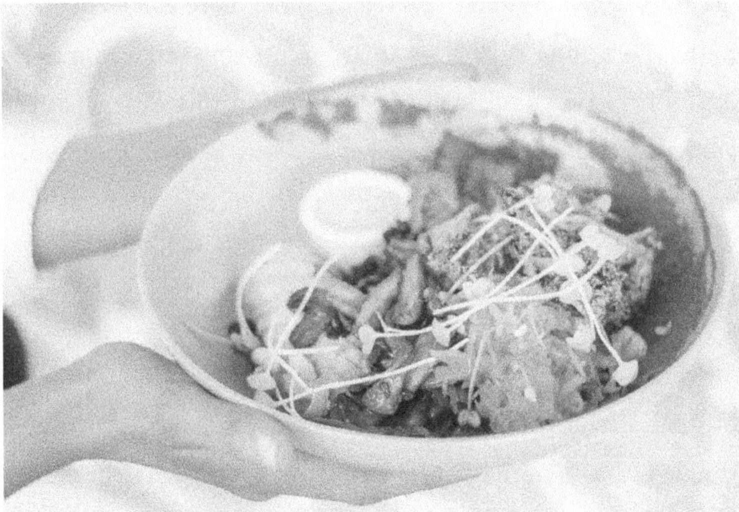

Fig. 10: Starting OMAD. Unsplash, by Maddi Bazzocco, 2018, https://unsplash.com/photos/qKbHvzXb85A/ Copyright 2018 by Maddi Bazzocco/Unsplash.

The OMAD method of intermittent fasting can potentially put you on a clearer path to health, happiness, and longevity. From start to finish, you have learned everything you need to know about the OMAD method—both good and bad—to determine whether it's right for you or not. If you decide to follow this method for the improvement of your health, then all you have to do is take that all-important first step.

In this book, we started off by learning all about intermittent fasting. As I have explained, this global trend isn't actually a diet. It's an eating pattern. Therefore, your focus won't be on the foods you will eat, but the time when you will eat your meals. It seems so simple and easy, but the more you learn about it, the more you realize how amazing intermittent fasting really is. To help you understand how and why this eating pattern works so well, we discussed what happens to your body when you eat and when you fast. The benefits of this eating pattern come during your fasting windows, the time when you aren't eating anything.

Speaking of benefits, we discussed all of the wonderful benefits of intermittent fasting in Chapter 2. As you have learned, this simple eating pattern offers a number of benefits to your health. If you can follow it correctly and stick with it long-term, IF can bring a lot of positive changes to your life. In Chapter 3, we discussed the most common methods of intermittent fasting. Although this eBook is focused on OMAD, learning about the other methods, and how to follow them can help you in your journey. This is especially true if you plan to start with a simpler method first before following OMAD.

In the next chapter, we started focusing on the One Meal A Day or OMAD method. Here, we defined what OMAD is and how to follow it. We also discussed the benefits of this specific method along with some initial tips for how to follow this extreme eating pattern. Here, I also introduced some of the downsides of OMAD, the other side that you should also know about so that you can truly determine if it is right for you. In Chapter 5, you were introduced to practical information about following the OMAD method. From starting slow, planning your meals, more tips, and knowing when to stop, this chapter should help you start your OMAD journey right away. It is in this chapter where I also shared a number of recipes for you to try out.

In the last chapter, we focused on the "dark side" of OMAD. Just like any other diet or eating pattern, OMAD also comes with its own risks. After all, it is one of the more extreme methods of intermittent fasting. If you think that you can follow OMAD without experiencing these side effects and risks, then it's time for you to begin. As I had promised you at the beginning of this book, I have shared everything I've learned as I embarked on my own OMAD journey. I started out wanting to overcome my insulin sensitivity and now, I have done that—and more.

As my final piece of advice for you, just remember to always listen to your body. If you think that you can succeed on OMAD while putting your health and safety first, then there is a very high chance that you will succeed. Thank you so much for taking the time to learn all about the OMAD method of intermittent fasting and how it can benefit your health. Now, as you finish this eBook, I wish you all the best on your OMAD journey. Hopefully, you will join us as one of the proponents of this extreme yet, highly beneficial eating pattern.

REFERENCES

30-Minute Coconut Curry. (n.d.). Retrieved from https://minimalistbaker.com/30-minute-coconut-curry/#_a5y_p=1531167

Allaf , M., Elghazaly , H., Mohamed , O. G., Fareen , F. K., Zaman , S., Salmasi , A. M., … Dehghan, A. (2019). Intermittent fasting for the prevention of cardiovascular disease. Retrieved from https://www.cochranelibrary.com/cdsr/doi/10.1002/14651858.CD013496/full

Anton, S. D., Moehl, K., Donahoo, W., & Marosi, K. (2017). Flipping the Metabolic Switch: Understanding and Applying the Health Benefits of Fasting: Flipping the Metabolic Switch. Retrieved from https://www.researchgate.net/publication/320733870_Flipping_the_Metabolic_Switch_Under

standing_and_Applying_the_Health_Benefits_of_Fasting_Flipping_the_Metabolic_Switch

Antoni, R., Johnston, K. L., Collins, A. L., & Robertson, M. D. (2014). The Effects of Intermittent Energy Restriction on Indices of Cardiometabolic Health. Retrieved from https://ibimapublishing.com/articles/ENDO/2014/459119/

Antunes, F., Erustes, A. G., Costa, A. J., Nascimento, A. C., Bincoletto, C., Ureshino, R. P., … Smaili, S. S. (2018). Autophagy and intermittent fasting: the connection for cancer therapy? Retrieved from https://www.ncbi.nlm.nih.gov/pmc/articles/PMC6257056/

Arnason, T. G., Bowen, M. W., & Mansell, K. D. (2017). Effects of intermittent fasting on health markers in those with type 2 diabetes: A pilot study. Retrieved from https://www.ncbi.nlm.nih.gov/pubmed/28465792

Azevedo, F. R. de, Ikeoka, D., & Caramelli, B. (2013). Effects of intermittent fasting on metabolism in men. Retrieved from https://www.sciencedirect.com/science/article/pii/S0104423013000213

Barnosky, A. R., Hoddy, K. K., Unterman, T. G., & Varady, K. A. (2014). Intermittent fasting vs daily calorie restriction for type 2 diabetes prevention: a review of human findings. Retrieved from https://www.ncbi.nlm.nih.gov/pubmed/24993615

Barnosky, A. R., Hoddy, K. K., Unterman, T. G., & Varady, K. A. (2014). Intermittent fasting vs daily calorie restriction for type 2 diabetes prevention: a review of human findings. Retrieved from https://www.sciencedirect.com/science/article/pii/S193152441400200X

Bauersfeld, S. P., Kessler, C. S., Wischnewsky, M., Jaensch, A., Steckhan, N., Stange, R., ... Michalsen, A. (2018). The effects of short-term fasting on quality of life and tolerance to chemotherapy in patients with breast and ovarian cancer: a randomized cross-over pilot study. Retrieved from https://bmccancer.biomedcentral.com/articles/10.1186/s12885-018-4353-2

Baum, I. (2019). What Is the OMAD Diet? Everything You Need to Know About This Extreme Intermittent Fasting Weight-Loss Plan. Retrieved from https://www.health.com/weight-loss/omad-diet

Bendix, A. (2019). 8 signs your intermittent fasting diet has become unsafe or unhealthy. Retrieved from https://www.businessinsider.com/signs-intermittent-fasting-unsafe-unhealthy-2019-7

Berardi, J. (2015). Intermittent Fasting: Whos It For? (And, if Its Not for You, What to Do Instead). Retrieved from https://www.huffpost.com/entry/intermittent-fasting-whos_b_6236712

Biswas , C. (2020). The One Meal A Day Diet (OMAD Diet) – How It Works, Health Benefits, And Safety. Retrieved from https://www.stylecraze.com/articles/one-meal-a-day-diet-the-ultimate-guide/

Blindow, A. (2019). Fasting: the body's natural stem cell therapy. Retrieved from https://www.intelligent.life/blog/fast-bodys-natural-stem-cell-therapy

Brusie, C. (2017). Is Eating One Meal a Day a Safe and Effective Way to Lose Weight? Retrieved from https://www.healthline.com/health/one-meal-a-day

Carstensen, M. (2018). Intermittent Fasting Helps Reverse Type 2 Diabetes in 3 Men: Study: Everyday Health. Retrieved from https://www.everydayhealth.com/type-2-diabetes/diet/intermittent-fasting-helps-reverse-type-2-diabetes-men-study/

Carter, S., Clifton, P. M., & Keogh, J. B. (2018). Effect of Intermittent vs Continuous Energy Restricted Diet on Glycemic Control in Type 2 Diabetes. Retrieved from https://jamanetwork.com/journals/jamanetworkopen/fullarticle/2688344

Chaix, A., Zarrinpar, A., Miu, P., & Panda, S. (2014). Time-Restricted Feeding Is a Preventative and Therapeutic Intervention against Diverse Nutritional Challenges. Retrieved from https://www.sciencedirect.com/science/article/pii/S1550413114004987?via=ihub

Chander, R. (2018). I Tried Extreme Fasting by Eating Once a Day — Here's What Happened. Retrieved from https://www.healthline.com/health/food-nutrition/one-meal-a-day-diet#1

Cole, W. (2019). OMAD Is The Biggest New Diet Trend For Decreasing Inflammation & Increasing Longevity. Retrieved from https://www.mindbodygreen.com/articles/omad-diet-what-it-is-if-its-safe-and-how-to-do-it

Common Dos and Don'ts of eating One Meal a Day (OMAD) - Times of India. (2019). Retrieved from https://timesofindia.indiatimes.com/life-style/health-fitness/diet/common-dos-and-donts-of-eating-one-meal-a-day-omad/articleshow/70805234.cms

Cording, J. (2019). Is the Secret to Losing Weight More About When You Eat Than What? Retrieved from https://www.shape.com/healthy-eating/diet-tips/potential-intermittent-fasting-benefits-not-worth-dieting-risks

de Cabo, R., & Mattson, M. P. (2019). Effects of Intermittent Fasting on Health, Aging, and Disease. Retrieved from https://www.gwern.net/docs/longevity/2019-decabo.pdf

de Groot, S., Pijl, H., van der Hoeven, J. J. M., & Kroep, J. R. (2019). Effects of short-term fasting on cancer treatment. Retrieved from https://jeccr.biomedcentral.com/articles/10.1186/s13046-019-1189-9

DeSantis, S. (2019). 30 Minute Vegan Breakfast Burritos. Retrieved from https://www.veggiesdontbite.com/30-minute-vegan-breakfast-burritos-minimalist-baker-everyday-cooking/

Denton, M. (2019). Anti-Aging Benefits of Intermittent Fasting. Retrieved from https://neurohacker.com/anti-aging-benefits-of-intermittent-fasting

Descamps, O., Riondel, J., Ducros, V., & Roussel, A.-M. (2005). Mitochondrial production of reactive oxygen species and incidence of age-associated lymphoma in OF1 mice: effect of alternate-day fasting. Retrieved from https://www.ncbi.nlm.nih.gov/pubmed/16126250

Diet Review: Intermittent Fasting for Weight Loss. (2019). Retrieved from https://www.hsph.harvard.edu/nutritionsource/healthy-weight/diet-reviews/intermittent-fasting/

Duan, W., Guo, Z., Jiang, H., Ware, M., Li, X.-J., & Mattson, M. P. (2003). Dietary restriction normalizes glucose metabolism and BDNF levels, slows disease progression, and increases survival in huntingtin mutant mice. Retrieved from https://www.ncbi.nlm.nih.gov/pmc/articles/PMC151440/

Easy Full English Keto Breakfast: KetoDiet Blog. (2020). Retrieved from https://ketodietapp.com/Blog/lchf/easy-full-english-keto-breakfast

Easy Pork Chops With Asparagus and Hollandaise: KetoDiet Blog. (2020). Retrieved from https://ketodietapp.com/Blog/lchf/easy-pork-chops-with-asparagus-and-hollandaise

Effects of Intermittent Fasting on Health, Aging, and Disease. (2020). Retrieved from https://www.crossfit.com/essentials/effects-of-intermittent-fasting-on-health-aging-and-disease

Eldridge, L. (2019). Can Intermittent Fasting Help Treat or Prevent Cancer? Retrieved from https://www.verywellhealth.com/intermittent-fasting-and-cancer-4772239

Exton, L. (2020). Quick Keto Salmon Power Bowl: KetoDiet Blog. Retrieved from https://ketodietapp.com/Blog/lchf/quick-keto-salmon-power-bowl

Fessenden, M. (2015). Mostly the Old And Ill Ate Breakfast Until the Rise of the Working Man. Retrieved from https://www.smithsonianmag.com/smart-news/mostly-old-and-ill-ate-breakfast-until-rise-working-man-180954041/

Fletcher, J. (2020). One meal a day: Health benefits and risks. Retrieved from https://www.medicalnewstoday.com/articles/320125

Fung, J. (2016). How to Renew Your Body: Fasting and Autophagy. Retrieved from https://www.dietdoctor.com/renew-body-fasting-autophagy

Furmli, S., Elmasry, R., Ramos, M., & Fung, J. (2017). Therapeutic use of intermittent fasting for people with type 2 diabetes as an alternative to insulin. Retrieved from https://casereports.bmj.com/content/2018/bcr-2017-221854.full

Gleeson, J. R. (2019). Intermittent Fasting: Is it Right for You? Retrieved from https://healthblog.uofmhealth.org/wellness-prevention/intermittent-fasting-it-right-for-you

Gleeson, J. R. (2019). Intermittent Fasting: Is it Right for You? Retrieved from https://healthblog.uofmhealth.org/wellness-prevention/intermittent-fasting-it-right-for-you

Goodrick, Charles L., I., K., D., A., M., Freeman, R., J., … Reynolds. (1983). Differential Effects of Intermittent Feeding and Voluntary Exercise on Body Weight and Lifespan in Adult Rats 1. Retrieved from https://academic.oup.com/geronj/article-abstract/38/1/36/570019

Gunnars, K. (2020). 6 Popular Ways to Do Intermittent Fasting. Retrieved from https://www.healthline.com/nutrition/6-ways-to-do-intermittent-fasting

Gunnars, K. (2017). How Intermittent Fasting Can Help You Lose Weight. Retrieved from https://www.healthline.com/nutrition/intermittent-fasting-and-weight-loss

Gunnars, K. (2016). 10 Evidence-Based Health Benefits of Intermittent Fasting. Retrieved from https://www.healthline.com/nutrition/10-health-benefits-of-intermittent-fasting

Haridy, R. (2019). Review of intermittent fasting research suggests broad health benefits. Retrieved from https://newatlas.

com/health-wellbeing/review-intermittent-fasting-research-health-benefits-johns-hopkins/

Hine, C., Harputlugil , E., Zhang , Y., Ruckenstuhl , C., Cheon Lee , B., Brace , L., ... Mitchell, J. R. (2014). Endogenous Hydrogen Sulfide Production Is Essential for Dietary Restriction Benefits. Retrieved from https://www.cell.com/cell/fulltext/S0092-8674(14)01525-6

How to start OMAD - One Meal a Day. (2018). Retrieved from https://desireepeeples.com/start-omad-one-meal-day/

Intermittent Fasting: 4 Different Types Explained. (2019). Retrieved from https://health.clevelandclinic.org/intermittent-fasting-4-different-types-explained/

Jarreau, P. B. (2018). Eating (Or rather, Fasting) Our Way to Rejuvenated Stem Cells? Retrieved from https://medium.com/lifeomic/eating-or-rather-fasting-our-way-to-rejuvenated-stem-cells-e4302a49e597

Johnson, J. B., Summer, W., Cutler, R. G., Martin, B., Hyun, D.-H., Dixit, V. D., ... Mattson, M. P. (2007). Alternate day calorie restriction improves clinical findings and reduces markers of oxidative stress and inflammation in overweight adults with moderate asthma. Retrieved from https://www.ncbi.nlm.nih.gov/pubmed/17291990/

Johnstone, A. (2015). Fasting for weight loss: an effective strategy or latest dieting trend? Retrieved from https://www.

ncbi.nlm.nih.gov/pubmed/25540982

Jordan , S., Tung , N., Casanova-Acebes , M., Chang , C., Cantoni , C., Zhang , D., ... Merad, M. (2019). Dietary Intake Regulates the Circulating Inflammatory Monocyte Pool. Retrieved from https://www.cell.com/cell/fulltext/S0092-8674(19)30850-5

Kerndt, P. R., Naughton, J. L., Driscoll, C. E., & Loxterkamp, D. A. (1982). Fasting: the history, pathophysiology and complications. Retrieved from https://www.ncbi.nlm.nih.gov/pubmed/6758355

Landsverk, G. (2019). Intermittent fasting may help slow aging and diseases like cancer and diabetes - even if you don't lose weight. Retrieved from https://www.insider.com/intermittent-fasting-slows-aging-cancer-diabetes-heart-disease-study-2019-12

Lee, C., Raffaghello, L., Brandhorst, S., Safdie, F. M., Bianchi, G., Martin-Montalvo, A., ... Longo, V. D. (2012). Fasting cycles retard growth of tumors and sensitize a range of cancer cell types to chemotherapy. Retrieved from https://www.ncbi.nlm.nih.gov/pubmed/22323820

Lee, J., Duan, W., Long, J. M., Ingram, D. K., & Mattson, M. P. (2000). Dietary restriction increases the number of newly generated neural cells, and induces BDNF expression, in the dentate gyrus of rats. Retrieved from https://www.ncbi.nlm.nih.gov/pubmed/11220789

Leech, J. (2019). 5 Stats That Show Why Intermittent Fasting is Powerful for Weight Loss. Retrieved from https://www.dietvsdisease.org/intermittent-fasting-is-powerful-for-weight-loss/

Leonard, J. (2020). 7 formas de hacer ayuno intermitente: Los mejores métodos. Retrieved from https://www.medicalnewstoday.com/articles/322293

Levy, J. (2018). Benefits of Autophagy, Plus How to Induce It. Retrieved from https://draxe.com/health/benefits-of-autophagy/

Li, L., Wang, Z., & Zuo, Z. (2013). Chronic intermittent fasting improves cognitive functions and brain structures in mice. Retrieved from https://www.ncbi.nlm.nih.gov/pmc/articles/PMC3670843/

Lindberg, S. (2018). Autophagy: What You Need to Know. Retrieved from https://www.healthline.com/health/autophagy

London, J. (2019, May 28). The Trendy OMAD Diet Has a Ton of Potentially Scary Side Effects. Retrieved from https://www.goodhousekeeping.com/health/diet-nutrition/a27506052/omad-diet/

Low-Carb Steak Taco Bowl: KetoDiet Blog. (2020). Retrieved from https://ketodietapp.com/Blog/lchf/low-carb-steak-taco-bowl

Magyar, O. (2017). Intermittent Fasting For Better Brain Health? Retrieved from https://neurotrition.ca/blog/intermittent-fasting-better-brain-health

Marosi, K., Moehl , K., Navas-Enamorado, I., Mitchell, S. J., Zhang, Y., Lehrmann , E., ... Mattson, M. P. (2018). Metabolic and molecular framework for the enhancement of endurance by intermittent food deprivation. Retrieved from https://www.fasebj.org/doi/10.1096/fj.201701378RR

Mattson, M. P., Moehl, K., Ghena, N., Schmaedick, M., & Cheng, A. (2018). Intermittent metabolic switching, neuroplasticity and brain health. Retrieved from https://www.ncbi.nlm.nih.gov/pubmed/29321682

Mattson, M. P. (2005). Energy intake, meal frequency, and health: a neurobiological perspective. Retrieved from https://www.ncbi.nlm.nih.gov/pubmed/16011467

McLeod, C. (2019). Intermittent fasting is trendy but dietitians warn against it. Retrieved from https://www.bodyandsoul.com.au/nutrition/nutrition-tips/the-6-people-who-shouldnt-try-intermittent-fasting-according-to-a-dietitian/news-story/ca97f74fc904811f4b78281824dea72c

Migala, J. (2020). 7 Types of Intermittent Fasting: Which Is Best for You?: Everyday Health. Retrieved from https://www.everydayhealth.com/diet-nutrition/diet/types-intermittent-fasting-which-best-you/

Mihaylova, M. M., Cheng, C.-W., Cao, A. Q., Tripathi, S., Mana, M. D., Bauer-Rowe, K. E., ... Yilmaz, Ö. H. (2018). Fasting Activates Fatty Acid Oxidation to Enhance Intestinal Stem Cell Function during Homeostasis and Aging. Retrieved from https://www.sciencedirect.com/science/article/pii/S1934590918301632

Moller, N., Vendelbo, M. H., Kampmann, U., Christensen, B., Madsen, M., Norrelund, H., & Jorgensen, J. O. (2009). Growth hormone and protein metabolism. Retrieved from https://www.ncbi.nlm.nih.gov/pubmed/19773097

Moro, T., Tinsley, G., Bianco, A., Marcolin, G., Pacelli, Q. F., Battaglia, G., ... Paoli, A. (2016). Effects of eight weeks of time-restricted feeding (16/8) on basal metabolism, maximal strength, body composition, inflammation, and cardiovascular risk factors in resistance-trained males. Retrieved from https://translational-medicine.biomedcentral.com/articles/10.1186/s12967-016-1044-0

Nørrelund, H., Nair, K. S., Jørgensen, J. O., Christiansen, J. S., & Møller, N. (2001). The protein-retaining effects of growth hormone during fasting involve inhibition of muscle-protein breakdown. Retrieved from https://www.ncbi.nlm.nih.gov/pubmed/11147801

O'Flanagan, C. H., Smith, L. A., McDonell, S. B., & Hursting, S. D. (2017). When less may be more: calorie restriction and response to cancer therapy. Retrieved from https://www.ncbi.nlm.nih.gov/pubmed/28539118

OMAD DIET: THE ULTIMATE GUIDE. (2019). Retrieved from https://omadmealplan.com/

Oppenheim, S. (2019). Is Intermittent Fasting Really The Healthiest Way To Eat? Not For Everyone. Retrieved from https://www.forbes.com/sites/serenaoppenheim/2019/01/24/is-intermittent-fasting-really-the-healthiest-way-to-eat-not-for-everyone/#276fd2d13606

Paddock, C. (2018). How fasting boosts exercise's effects on endurance. Retrieved from https://www.medicalnewstoday.com/articles/321056

Park, M. (2010). Nearing 50, Renaissance jock Herschel Walker breaks fitness rules. Retrieved from http://edition.cnn.com/2010/HEALTH/10/11/herschel.fitness.martial.arts/index.html

Pattillo, A. (2019). The Truth Behind What Intermittent Fasting Does to Your Body. Retrieved from https://www.inverse.com/article/57625-what-intermittent-fasting-actually-does-to-your-body

Pawlowski, A. (2019). What is the OMAD diet? Learn how the one-meal-a-day plan works. Retrieved from https://www.today.com/health/what-omad-diet-learn-how-one-meal-day-diet-works-t146204

Permanente, K. (n.d.). How our bodies turn food into energy. Retrieved from https://wa.kaiserpermanente.org/healthAndWellness?item=/common/healthAndWellness/conditions/diabetes/foodProcess.html

Pleimling, A. (2017). Trendy or troublesome? Get the facts on intermittent fasting. Retrieved from https://www.allinahealth.org/healthysetgo/nourish/trendy-or-troublesome-the-facts-on-intermittent-fasting

Phillips, M. C. L. (2019). Fasting as a Therapy in Neurological Disease. Retrieved from https://www.ncbi.nlm.nih.gov/pmc/articles/PMC6836141/

Presto, G. (2017). Is Intermittent Fasting Right For You? Retrieved from https://www.bornfitness.com/intermittent-fasting/

Research on intermittent fasting shows health benefits. (2020, February 27). Retrieved from https://www.nia.nih.gov/news/research-intermittent-fasting-shows-health-benefits

Researchers discover that fasting reduces inflammation and improves chronic inflammatory diseases. (2019). Retrieved from https://medicalxpress.com/news/2019-08-fasting-inflammation-chronic-inflammatory-diseases.html

Ries, J. (2020). This Is Your Body On Intermittent Fasting. Retrieved from https://www.huffpost.com/entry/body-intermittent-fasting_l_5e0a3220c5b6b5a713b22dcb?

guccounter=1&guce_referrer=
aHR0cHM6Ly93d3cuZ29vZ2xlLmNvbS8&guce_referrer_sig=
AQAAAC-
HM3NWPXeuZI89BsKO_6IpI8l9andTLuWwBQJfgG-
AsuIWgujK_56SnSe6nwtztpxQJ50POffVrpAasbAvte9Zq5Z31
m4DPBrmQfjl-gS1ahKuyRQNZApPT-
6VAiMjRY5SqN1g6Vcfx_jg2BiwVYsMz8SklicgTXv6h1SZI-GS

Rinzler, C. A., & DeVault, K. (n.d.). The Human Digestion Process (or, What Happens after You Eat Food). Retrieved from https://www.dummies.com/education/science/biology/the-human-digestion-process-or-what-happens-after-you-eat-food/

Rose, E. (2020). OMAD: What is One Meal a Day Fasting, and Should You Try It? Retrieved from https://www.bulletproof.com/diet/intermittent-fasting/omad-one-meal-a-day-diet/

Rumi Quote: "Fasting is the first principle of medicine; fast and see the strength of the spirit reveal itself.". (n.d.). Retrieved from https://quotefancy.com/quote/904488/Rumi-Fasting-is-the-first-principle-of-medicine-fast-and-see-the-strength-of-the-spirit

Save, K. (2019). What really happens to your body during intermittent fasting. Retrieved from https://www.bodyandsoul.com.au/diet/diets/what-really-happens-to-your-body-during-intermittent-fasting/news-story/92cdbf27507d9fa3afe30eaab3172b5e

Scher, B. (2020). What You Need to Know About OMAD. Retrieved from https://www.dietdoctor.com/intermittent-fasting/omad

Schmidt, M. (2020). What Science Says About the Weight-Loss Potential of 'OMAD' Fasting - The One-Meal-a-Day Diet. Retrieved from https://www.discovermagazine.com/health/what-science-says-about-the-weight-loss-potential-of-omad-fasting-the-one

Seimon, R. V., Roekenes, J. A., Zibellini, J., Zhu, B., Gibson, A. A., Hills, A. P., ... Sainsbury, A. (2015). Do intermittent diets provide physiological benefits over continuous diets for weight loss? A systematic review of clinical trials. Retrieved from https://www.sciencedirect.com/science/article/abs/pii/S0303720715300800?via=ihub

Sigurdsson, A. F. (2020). Intermittent Fasting and Health – The Scientific Evidence. Retrieved from https://www.docsopinion.com/intermittent-fasting

Sisson, M. (2020). 7 Tips and Considerations for Eating One Meal a Day. Retrieved from https://www.marksdailyapple.com/7-tips-and-considerations-for-eating-one-meal-a-day/

Sogawa, H., & Kubo, C. (2000). Influence of short-term repeated fasting on the longevity of female (NZB×NZW)F1 mice. Retrieved from https://www.sciencedirect.com/science/article/abs/pii/S0047637400001093

Southard, L. (2020). What is OMAD diet: Why eating one meal a day isn't recommended by experts. Retrieved from https://www.insider.com/what-is-omad-diet

Stieg, C. (2019). Is The OMAD Diet The New Intermittent Fasting? Retrieved from https://www.refinery29.com/en-us/eating-one-meal-a-day-diet-trend

Stote, K. S., Baer, D. J., Spears, K., Paul, D. R., Harris, G. K., Rumpler, W. V., ... Mattson, M. P. (2007). A controlled trial of reduced meal frequency without caloric restriction in healthy, normal-weight, middle-aged adults. Retrieved from https://www.ncbi.nlm.nih.gov/pmc/articles/PMC2645638/

Sweet Potato Taco Bowl. (2019). Retrieved from https://www.mykitchenlove.com/sweet-potato-taco-bowl/

Tello, M. (2020). Intermittent fasting: Surprising update. Retrieved from https://www.health.harvard.edu/blog/intermittent-fasting-surprising-update-2018062914156

Templeman, I., Gonzalez, J. T., Thompson, D., & Betts, J. A. (2020). The role of intermittent fasting and meal timing in weight management and metabolic health. Retrieved from https://www.ncbi.nlm.nih.gov/pubmed/31023390

Templeton, L. (2019). Intermittent fasting can help ease metabolic syndrome. Retrieved from https://www.medicalnewstoday.com/articles/327247

The Dangers of Intermittent Fasting. (2019). Retrieved from https://centerfordiscovery.com/blog/the-dangers-of-intermittent-fasting/

The OMAD Diet: Is Having One Meal A Day Effective? (2020). Retrieved from https://betterme.world/articles/omad-diet/

The Warrior Diet: Review and Beginner's Guide. (2018). Retrieved from https://www.healthline.com/nutrition/warrior-diet-guide

Tinsley, G. M., & La Bounty, P. M. (2015). Effects of intermittent fasting on body composition and clinical health markers in humans. Retrieved from https://academic.oup.com/nutritionreviews/article/73/10/661/1849182

Top 10 Tips for OMAD - Tips for One Meal a Day Diet. (2019). Retrieved from http://siimland.com/top-10-tips-for-omad-tips-for-one-meal-a-day-diet/

Varady, K. A., & Hellerstein, M. K. (2007). Alternate-day fasting and chronic disease prevention: a review of human and animal trials. Retrieved from https://www.ncbi.nlm.nih.gov/pubmed/17616757?dopt=Abstract

Varady, K. A., Bhutani, S., Church, E. C., & Klempel, M. C. (2009). Short-term modified alternate-day fasting: a novel dietary strategy for weight loss and cardioprotection in obese adults. Retrieved from https://www.ncbi.nlm.nih.gov/pubmed/19793855

Varady, K. A. (2011). Intermittent versus daily calorie restriction: which diet regimen is more effective for weight loss? Retrieved from https://www.ncbi.nlm.nih.gov/pubmed/21410865

Weindruch, R., & Sohal, R. S. (1997). Seminars in medicine of the Beth Israel Deaconess Medical Center. Caloric intake and aging. Retrieved from https://www.ncbi.nlm.nih.gov/pmc/articles/PMC2851235/

West, H. (2016). Does Intermittent Fasting Boost Your Metabolism? Retrieved from https://www.healthline.com/nutrition/intermittent-fasting-metabolism

What happens to the food we eat? - (Food and Body Function). (n.d.). Retrieved from http://apjcn.nhri.org.tw/server/info/books-phds/books/foodfacts/html/maintext/main3a.html

Wilkinson, M. J., Manoogian, E. N. C., Zadourian, A., Navlakha, S., Lo, H., Fakhouri, S., ... Taub, P. R. (2019). Ten-Hour Time-Restricted Eating Reduces Weight, Blood Pressure, and Atherogenic Lipids in Patients with Metabolic Syndrome. Retrieved from https://www.cell.com/cell-metabolism/fulltext/S1550-4131(19)30611-4

Zahid, U. (2019). (Ultimate Guide) All You Need to Know About OMAD Diet. Retrieved from https://ashrafchaudhryblog.com/omad-diet/

Zarrinpar, A., Chaix, A., Yooseph, S., & Panda, S. (2014). Diet and feeding pattern affect the diurnal dynamics of the gut microbiome. Retrieved from https://www.ncbi.nlm.nih.gov/pubmed/25470548

Zhang, J., Zhan, Z., Li, X., Xing, A., Jiang, C., Chen, Y., ... An, L. (2017). Intermittent Fasting Protects against Alzheimer's Disease Possible through Restoring Aquaporin-4 Polarity. Retrieved from https://www.ncbi.nlm.nih.gov/pmc/articles/PMC5712566/

WATER FASTING

HOW TO LOSE WEIGHT FAST, INCREASE MENTAL CLARITY, HEAL YOUR BODY, & ACTIVATE AUTOPHAGY WITH WATER FASTING

INTRODUCTION

"By fasting, the body learns to obey the soul; by praying, the soul learns to command the body."

— WILLIAM SECKER (WELLMAN, 2015)

In this age of constant stress, anxiety, and increasing levels of chronic illness, many of us seek ways to repair and, hopefully, reverse the damage we have done to our bodies through living this lifestyle. While 20 years ago, the World Health Organization deemed undernutrition or starvation to be the most pressing global health issue, today we are faced with quite the opposite. Overnutrition, leading to obesity, has become the primary health concern globally, even in underdeveloped countries. Obesity is a major risk factor in many chronic diseases including cardiovascular disease, diabetes, and hypertension. The shift in this global health dynamic has led to the emergence of many fad diets and self-appointed experts who will promise you immediate, dramatic, and sustained weight loss with no scientific data or social proof to back up their claims. Sadly, these fad diets can often do more harm than good in the long term. While you may lose weight, because these new and unproven diets and eating plans are often the unscientific brainchild of nonprofessionals, you will never know what long-term damage may be done to your body. The other side of the coin is that even if these fad diets work, they will only help you lose weight, and you will not see any other overall health benefits. This is where fasting is different.

As an age-old practice, fasting has thousands of years of scientific backing and social proof behind it. Possibly one of the most well-known religious and spiritual connections to fasting is the celebration of Ramadan, which is a fasting period practiced by Muslims. Ramadan fast participants have been shown to have an improved immune response during this time, indicating the positive impact of fasting on the body. Fasting is a lifestyle that will not only help you to lose weight safely but also provide you with a huge number of other health benefits. Although fasting has its roots in ancient times, it has, more recently, gained popularity as a weight-loss and health improvement practice. This sudden surge in public interest has also led to a lot of misinformation, and it is important to clarify its roots and uses, and the actual scientific basis of how fasting works, in order for it to be properly understood and used to its greatest effect. Thankfully, fasting is the darling of the research community, as it consistently provides measurable results in clinical settings, so there is plenty of data and information to work with in making the decision as to whether fasting is right for you.

It is very likely that you already have a good idea of what fasting is, but I would like to define the concept for you from the outset for purposes of clarity. Fasting is essentially the voluntary restriction of the consumption of food to certain time periods. Fasting is not starvation, as this term implies being forced to withhold food, and it also implies that some form of damage is done to the body. Fasting is quite the opposite. When carried out correctly, fasting, as part of a lifestyle, can not only help you lose weight but also trigger and accelerate natural processes within your body that promote greater overall physical, mental, and emotional health. Our bodies are not built to be in a constantly fed state, and when we do withhold food from ourselves, our bodies react positively. Hormones are released into the bloodstream that help to maintain our glucose levels, regulate our appetite, improve our metabolic response, and even impact the nervous system.

Fasting also triggers a natural process within our body called autophagy. Autophagy is our body's way of cleaning out old, dead, and damaged cells and using that cellular material to create new, healthy cells. The process starts when we are born and occurs at a high rate in our bodies when we are young. This is why children and younger people tend to heal quicker than older people. As we age, the process of autophagy starts to naturally slow in our bodies, again resulting in the slower healing of older people from disease and injury. In 2016, Japanese cellular biologist Yoshinori Ohsumi won a Nobel Prize for his research into autophagy, which revealed an excellent method of accelerating the process no matter your age—fasting. During his study, Ohsumi found that when the body is in a fasted state, autophagy is triggered, and when it is in a fed state, it slows down (The Nobel Prize in Physiology or Medicine, 2016). This discovery has contributed to our understanding of exactly how fasting provides all of the health benefits that it does. Interestingly, the research is so compelling that pharmaceutical companies are now trying to develop a synthetic trigger for autophagy. This seems rather counterintuitive, though, as if there is a natural way to kickstart this self-healing process. There is no reason to introduce a chemical method which can only have negative side effects.

The specific focus of this book is water fasting. If you have already looked into fasting, it is perhaps important to explain how water fasting is different from other types of fasting, such as intermittent fasting. When you practice water fasting, you do not eat at all. You only consume water in order to ensure that you remain hydrated and to help your body expel the toxins and waste that the accelerated autophagy process creates. Those who practice intermittent fasting will have eating windows and fasting windows within a 24-hour period, but with water fasting, the only thing you consume is water. Water fasting is shown to have significant benefits including weight loss, the promotion of autophagy, the stabilization of blood pressure, and the improvement of the body's response to hormones like insulin and leptin.

Having explained the benefits of this protocol to you, I think it is also important for me to explain to you how I discovered water fasting and how it has been beneficial for me. I started suffering from insulin resistance in my early 20s. It affected my weight, it increased my risk of diabetes, and I thought I had no choice but to go on the medications that the doctors prescribed at such an early age. Regardless of the pharmaceutical and diet interventions, my insulin sensitivity did not improve enough to give me back the life I had previously known. This had a huge impact on me emotionally, and I felt as though my youth was being snatched away from me. Motivated to make healthier life choices, I started researching holistic and alternative practices when I turned 30. This was when I came across intermittent fasting and even more importantly–water fasting. I started incorporating both into my routine, also focusing on mindfulness, meditation, and the selection of the right foods. In time, I was able t0 lose 50 pounds. My insulin sensitivity improved so much that my doctors cleared me to stop taking medications.

Years on and in good health, I have summed up all of my research and my personal practices in two books–*Water*

Fasting and *One Meal a Day Intermittent Fasting*. I created these books with a lot of love and compassion for others, hoping that this information will help others to transform their lives and benefit from the health improvements hidden in such simple practices.

You have likely purchased this book because you have physical issues that you need to address. Such issues may include an excess weight that you need to lose, dealing with chronic illness, or simply aiming to increase your longevity and improve your cognitive functioning. My goal for you is that by the end of this book, you will have gained the knowledge and skills required to implement water fasting as a lifestyle solution to these health issues and that you will be confident enough to proceed and succeed.

Knowledge is absolutely vital in ensuring a successful water fast as it is not just the fast itself that must be specifically structured but also the prefast period and the postfast period. All three of these periods are equally important in water fasting, and that is, perhaps, one of the things that makes water fasting so different from other forms of fasting. Whereas in other forms of fasting there is definitely focus on easing out of the fast, this is emphasized greatly in water fasting. There is also significant emphasis on the prefast period and preparations for the fast in the run-up to it. If you have tried other types of fasting before, you will find that it is these preparations that make water fasting far more effective and easier to manage.

I would like *Water Fasting: How to Lose Weight Fast, Increase Mental Clarity, Heal Your Body, & Activate Autophagy With Water Fasting,* to be an all-around resource for you in your water fasting journey. It will provide you with every tool you need and answer every question you may have about water fasting. Your journey with water fasting is about to begin.

1

THE HISTORY OF WATER FASTING

Water fasting has been practiced since the first written record of humanity and probably even before we had the capability to produce written documents. The sudden, recent popularity of various forms of fasting may give people the mistaken impression that it is a new practice. The history of water fasting is very important to understand, though, because it reflects its synchronicity with the way our bodies have evolved and takes us back to a time when we ate in a way that was beneficial to our bodies. Water fasting was originally a very common practice which aided ancient civilizations in carrying out certain activities. Our ancient ancestors understood that while certain foods are excellent from a medicinal perspective, some of the most significant healing happens in the body when we are not eating.

FASTING THROUGHOUT THE AGES

Our ancient ancestors did not live in the constantly fed state that has become our custom in today's world. Until the first Agricultural Revolution (circa 10,000 BC), food was only available when sought out through hunting or gathering. As such, human beings would eat only when food was available, and the rest of the time they survived in a fasted state with water as hydration. It is this initial state of occasional eating that, in fact, helped us to evolve the internal energy system we use today. Our bodies started to store energy so that we could burn it when we needed to. In the Neolithic Age, man began to settle down and understand the value of farming crops and animals in one place. At this point, man began to slowly change his eating habits but still continued to eat, largely, when food was available. When the second Agricultural Revolution dawned in the 18th century, crop and livestock farming became mechanized. Even after the Agricultural Age, when food did become more readily available, civilizations still maintained a predominantly fasted state and acknowledged the usefulness of fasting in promoting good health.

Prior to the acknowledgement that fasting has an impact on our physical health, it was used predominantly for spiritual purposes as a form of soul cleansing or spiritual journey. Even at that time, though, healers and those involved in the study of medicine understood that the mind and body are connected, and what is good for one must ultimately be good for the other.

Probably one of the most famous pioneers of medicine, the ancient Greek physician, Hippocrates, included in his writings that fasting enabled the body to heal itself. He indicated that, in his opinion, to eat when one is sick is to feed your illness. This concept of not eating when we are ill is, of course, a very natural instinct within our body. Animals, too, will stop eating when they are particularly ill. Today, we take this as an indication that it's time to rush off to the doctor, but in ancient times, it was understood that this was simply an indication that the body was beginning to heal itself. Another well-known ancient Greek, the mathematician Pythagoras, who only took on disciples if they were capable of fasting for a set period, also wrote about fasting in his texts, with philosophers Plato and Aristotle also weighing in on the topic. Fasting was therefore a very popular practice in Ancient Greece and also emerged as a central practice in Ayurvedic medicine, which is still popular today and involves healing the mind, body, and soul as a unit rather than separate entities.

Greece's ancient relationship with fasting would rear its head many centuries later when Mediterranean diet guru Dr. Ancel Keys decided that it was this diet that led to the exceptional levels of health and longevity in the people of Crete. It was soon pointed out to him, though, that these same people had also practiced fasting for many generations.

Ancient warriors would use fasting during battle as they were unable to eat for long periods while they marched or fought, so they would hold off until they were camped out between battles or they had returned home in order to celebrate with a feast. It was also common for soldiers to fast before battles in order to ensure their bodies were in peak condition and that they were mentally aware. Fasting was also used as a coming of age ritual and to avoid natural catastrophes and angered idols.

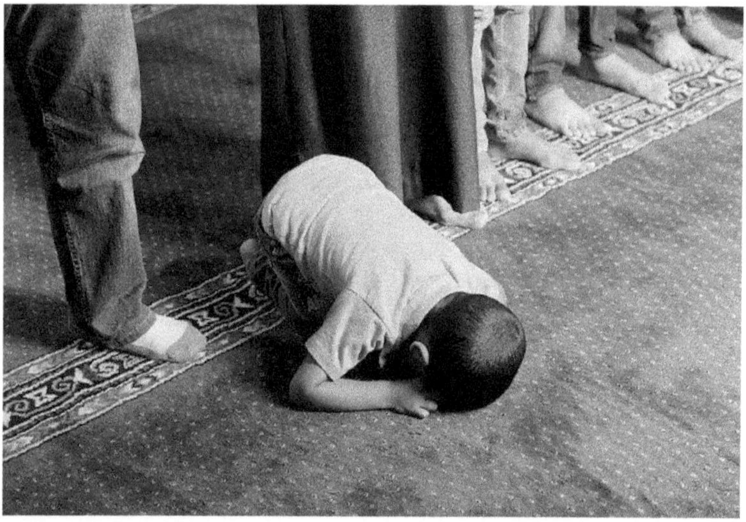

Most major world religions practice a form of fasting as part of their traditions, with the one exception being Zoroastrianism. The fast during the holy month of Ramadan, practiced by followers of Islam, lasts from sunrise to sunset each day. Water and other liquids are forbidden during the fasting period in Ramadan. Due to its extended nature, this religious fast is the most studied of all fasts and has shown that binging at the end of a fast can negate all of the good done during the fast.

Buddhists will often only eat in the morning and practice a daily fast that extends after this meal through to the next day. Buddhists also include water fasts as part of their rituals for several days or even weeks. Greek Orthodox Christians also include fasting as part of their traditions on up to 200 separate days of the year. Judaism also has several fasting days within its traditional calendar, including Yom Kippur, and Roman Catholics fast for 40 days during Lent. During the Renaissance, physicians and medical scholars wrote significantly about fasting, with one great healer, Paracelcus, referring to fasting as "the physician within." (Short History of Fasting, 2017). In reading these ancient scripts, it seems clear that even at this time they understood the great healing mechanism that is activated by fasting. Women in history seem to have linked religion or spirituality and fasting far more than men, with a practice being carried out which encouraged the refusal of food for long periods in order to prove one's purity of body and soul. A 14th century English mystic, Julian of Norwich, claimed to use fasting as a means of communication with Christ. For ancient spiritualists, it seemed that when we are able to free our minds from the binds of hunger and thoughts of food, our minds become clearer, and we are more able to focus on becoming deeply spiritually aware.

Quite separately from religion, fasting spawned itself into a method of political statement, such as that used by Mahatma Gandhi in 17 fasts he conducted in his quest to free India from colonial rule. Gandhi's longest fast lasted 21 days. The way in which Gandhi used fasts as a method of social protest is quite interesting. Another term for what he was doing is, of course, a "hunger strike," but when fasting was used by Gandhi, it was not used as a weapon to force others to give in to his demands as he "withered away" before their eyes. Mahatma Gandhi used fasting in his daily life as a means of spiritual purification, and it was not uncommon for him to fast outside of the public eye. It seems that although the public may have seen these protests as hunger strikes, it was more a way of Gandhi proving his persistence and refreshing his mind in order to continue pursuing the justice and freedom he sought for his country. Gandhi's roots as a traditional Hindi, his preference for nonviolent protests, and his vegetarianism all seem to blend well with him practicing fasting as a lifestyle rather than just a method of protest.

The Suffragettes was another famous group of social protesters who used fasting as a means of getting their point across, although for this group, it seemed far more like a hunger strike than a fast for health or spiritual reasons. The Suffragettes was a group of women in the 1900s who campaigned for the rights of women to vote. When imprisoned for their acts of protest, the women would undertake hunger strikes to force prison officials to release them. One particular Suffragette, Marion Wallace-Dunlop, began to refuse all food while imprisoned, and when a prison doctor examined her and asked her what she would eat, she replied, "My determination" (Purvis, 2009). Wallace-Dunlop was released after fasting for 91 hours as prison officials were afraid that she would die on their watch, which would result in a public uproar. If the prison officials had known anything about fasting, they would have realized that she could have continued for far longer than 91 hours as long as she had water. It is, perhaps, these hunger-strike-type fasts which have imprinted themselves on our memories as a collective and driven the narrative that choosing not to eat is somehow an act of desperation.

One of America's founding fathers, Benjamin Franklin, was a great supporter of the idea that the best medicine for most conditions is to rest and fast.

When something is known to work well, it is often skewed and manipulated to suit the needs of those with nefarious intentions, and fasting is no different. A rather dark part of the history of fasting occurred in 1912, when a self-proclaimed doctor, Linda Burfield Hazzard, formed a cult of sorts in Minnesota. The woman based her teachings and healings around the concept of fasting, but instead of using the practice to benefit people, she used it to harm them. It is believed that at least 40 patients died at the hands of Hazzard after she refused the people, who were already in very poor health, any food or water for several weeks. Thankfully, this horrendous act was a one-off occurrence, and after Hazzard's death in 1938, fasting started to move into its own as a truly beneficial health practice.

The benefits of fasting, including water fasting, were explored further in the 19th Century. The US saw a movement begin called the National Hygiene Movement, which supported therapeutic fasting for the treatment of illnesses, with the opening of a clinic by Dr. Herbert Shelton in 1928. Shelton promoted alternative medicine, including the use of fasting as a healing mechanism. He was also a vegetarian and promoter of raw eating. Shelton reported that he had helped over 40,000 patients overcome their physical ailments through fasting at his clinic (Short History of Fasting, 2017).

At the same time, in the UK, water fasts were being promoted as part of that country's own alternative medicine movement, called Nature Cure. Clinics sprung up across the United Kingdom, and some still exist in different forms today. The clinics advocated therapeutic fasting and had significant success in treating a wide variety of physical ailments. As pharmaceuticals became more widely used and people started to understand that they could take a drug for their ailments, these clinics started to wane in popularity (Short History of Fasting, 2017).

WATER FASTING IN THE PRESENT DAY

Today, different parts of the world seem to have held on to fasting more vehemently than others. Europe and the United Kingdom, specifically, have many fasting clinics that operate to this day. Tom Greenfield is a naturopath who heads up a fasting clinic in Canterbury, England. It is an offshoot of the original "Nature Cure" clinics, and Greenfield says that he still has patients that fasted at the original clinic. Greenfield admits that as medication has become more prevalent, fasting has become less popular, even in areas where it was once the go-to practice, but the patients that he has been treating for years understand and value the power of fasting and have continued its practice throughout their lives.

In Germany, therapeutic fasting is still very popular even today and is offered at various clinics across the country. German health insurance companies even work with hospitals to fund fasting promotion weeks. European fasting vacations are even popular at specialized spas and centers. The German people call fasting part of their "naturheilkunde," or natural health practice, and medical doctors in Germany are well known for prescribing fasting as complementary therapy for patients.

In the present day, we seem to have come full circle, in that we have started to acknowledge that medicating ourselves is not necessarily the best long-term solution. All chemical drugs, after all, have some form of negative side effect and can ultimately do more harm than good. It is this acknowledgement, in part, that has led us back to a focus on a natural way of doing things, including water fasting. The concepts of fasting and water fasting, in their growing popularity, have been adopted by many real experts and some pseudoexperts, who may make wild claims and promises that cannot necessarily be fulfilled. It is therefore vital to enter into water fasting armed with knowledge so that you understand what is possible and how the data backs up those claims. One of the major shifts in how we fast now compared to how we used to fast is that we are no longer able to fast as long as the ancient Greeks did, for instance. This is because of the nature of the world we live in. The many pollutants and stresses that exist in our modern world have made modern man constitutionally weaker and therefore unable to complete the extreme periods of fasting which were possible for ancient man. This doesn't mean that we can't bring ourselves into a state that is closer to where we began, though. Each time we fast, we shift our bodies further away from the unhealthy state that has become the norm for us today.

In preparing to start water fasting, it is important to understand how to do so safely and also what results you can expect. In the chapters that follow, I will provide you with actionable steps, evidence, and science-backed information regarding water fasting, and a guide to experiencing all of the available benefits. Be sure to take a slow read through the information that follows and absorb and understand the facts. In order to learn, we must think critically and actively question the information that we are given. It is insufficient to enter water fasting thinking that it's just about not eating. That very basic understanding does not help you to achieve the results you desire. In order to be successful in water fasting, you must understand precisely how the process works in your body so that you can prepare properly, fast correctly, and, most importantly, break your fast correctly.

2

WHO CAN DO A WATER FAST?

Before deciding whether to start water fasting, it is important to understand the situations and circumstances in which one should not practice water fasting. Although it is a generally safe practice, there are certain people for whom water fasting is not the best choice. In many of these situations, once the circumstances have resolved themselves, you can then proceed with water fasting. If any doubt is present as to whether water fasting is a safe option for you, always consult a doctor, and continue to gain factual information about fasting until you are 100% convinced that it is right for you. Starting a practice like fasting with doubts is not setting yourself up for success, and really, when it comes to your health, you should never do anything that you have a single doubt about. Thankfully, it is quite easy to differentiate between those who can attempt fasting safely and those who should stay away from the practice. Nothing is ever concrete, though, when we talk about the individuality of health; therefore, there is no replacement for understanding and listening to your body and giving it what it needs.

BEFORE YOU DECIDE

If you have never water fasted before, it is a good idea to visit your doctor before you start for a full health assessment. This will rule out any underlying issues that you may be experiencing which could be aggravated by water fasting. Anyone who suffers from a chronic medical condition or is on chronic medication should carefully consider whether water fasting is right for them. Also, be sure to start slowly and build your way up to longer fasting periods. It may be an interesting exercise to have a range of tests done before you start fasting. This way, you can do your own personal study of exactly how water fasting affects your cholesterol, blood sugar, blood pressure, and other body measurements.

All beginners should start with a fast that is no longer than 24 hours. Every individual is different, and the longer fasts are simply not suitable for some people. You will already gain great benefit from the initial 24-hour fast, so if a longer fast is not suitable for you, then you are not losing out too significantly on further benefits. It is important to listen to your body and be really aware of how you are feeling both during and after fasting. Successful fasting is a fine line between pushing your body into a natural state that it may not be used to and ensuring that you, as an individual, are staying within your limitations. By starting with a shorter fast and working your way up, you can find your "sweet spot" in which you are receiving the greatest benefit and also maintaining awareness of your body's limitations. It is important to recognize the difference between physical and mental limitations and to understand that both are important; however, mental or emotional limitations are easier to push through than physical limitations.

POSSIBLE RISKS

If water fasting is not done correctly, it can result in a range of physical risks presenting, and it is important to understand what these risks could be and how to avoid them. Water fasting consists of three stages—prefast, during the fast, and post fast—if any of those stages are incorrectly carried out, there are risks that can result. This is why knowledge and deep understanding of the practice and its physical impact on the body is so important before starting.

Dehydration

Dehydration is one of the most obvious risks to water fasting. Although you are supposed to take in water during your fast, it is not uncommon for people to only take in the same amount of water they would when they are not fasting, and this is where the problem comes in. About 30% of the fluid we take in daily actually comes from our food, so when we are fasting, we are already at a 30% fluid deficit from the outset. The other consideration is that most people do not drink enough water under normal circumstances, and although this may not lead to chronic dehydration when we are not fasting, it may become a problem when we do. Our ordinary eight glasses per day of water should therefore increase to at least 12 glasses per day when we are fasting to avoid dehydration.

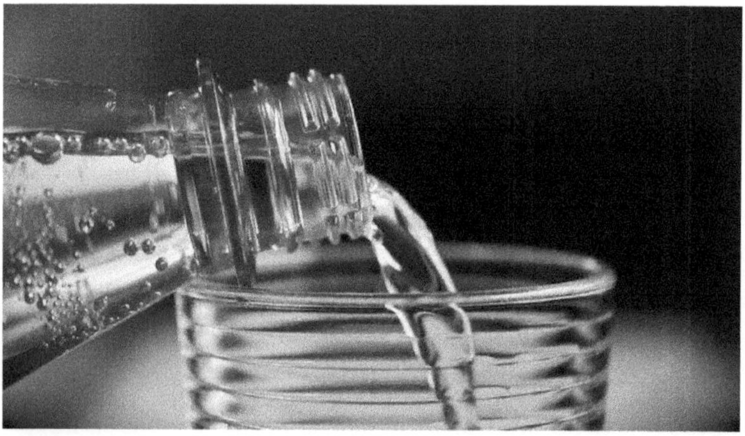

When Muslim people prepare for Ramadan (which is a dry fast), they will consume large amounts of water beforehand to ensure that they are sufficiently hydrated. They will also avoid taking part in any high-energy tasks which may result in a loss of hydration. Although Ramadan is a dry fast for religious reasons, there are those who believe that fasting for health reasons should involve no food or liquids by mouth during the fast period. Not drinking any fluid while fasting puts you at a far higher risk of doing damage to your body than water fasting or intermittent fasting and is not recommended for health or weight loss purposes. The side effects of a dry fast are also far more severe as water helps to relieve hunger, headaches, and aids the excretion of toxins through urination and sweating. During dry fasts, urination decreases significantly, which can cause kidney damage as well as urinary tract infections.

If you are water fasting and find that your urinary output has decreased significantly, increase your water intake immediately to avoid any of the added risks.

If you are a smoker and also wanting to attempt fasting, you will need to pay added attention to your water intake. Smoking cigarettes dehydrates the body, and smoking while fasting really defeats the purpose as you are continually adding toxins to a system that is trying to rid itself of toxins.

Nutrient Deficiencies

Another very common risk factor when fasting is not consuming the correct amount of nutrients. Our best source of nutrients is always food, and when we are fasting, we are not taking in those nutrients. Deficiencies can lead to a wide array of health issues. In order to avoid this, before you start fasting look for a good quality, wide-spectrum multivitamin supplement. Most of these supplements will be zero calorie but make sure you check the box or pack to ensure that they are indeed not going to interfere with your fast. Some people can feel nauseated when taking vitamin supplements on an empty stomach so be sure to drink the tablet with plenty of water to fill your stomach.

Taking supplements while fasting can also cause your blood sugar to drop significantly, which will further reduce your energy levels and increase brain fog. Some supplements may increase your insulin levels and take you out of the fat-burning process. There are also supplements that cannot work without food, and if you take them while fasting, they will pass directly through your body. The wisest option may be to discuss supplements with your doctor before starting fasting; otherwise, finding the right supplement may become a trial-and-error project and waste significant time. You will need to avoid supplements that are fat soluble as these must be taken with food. Other supplements, though, work best when taken with others, including vitamin A, D, and K. Vitamins B and C are water soluble and therefore can be taken without food. L-tyrosine is an excellent amino acid supplement which works well on a fast and helps to improve your mood and cognitive function. The following supplements are fat soluble and can only be taken with food:

- vitamins e, a, d, and k
- iodine
- magnesium
- chromium
- zinc and copper

When we are water fasting, supplements can help us to avoid nutrient deficiencies, but when we are eating normally again, it is far healthier to get our nutrients from the food we eat. If we are eating a well-balanced diet and we don't suffer from any abnormal absorption issues, then we really shouldn't need supplements. Understanding which nutrients we may be missing can be a bit of a guessing game without carrying out a battery of blood tests. Other than ensuring that your diet consists of a wide variety of fresh, whole foods, there are also some physical signs that you can look out for that are your body's way of telling you that you are experiencing a deficiency.

Iron is probably one of the most common nutrient deficiencies, and this results in chronic tiredness, a weakened immune system, general weakness in the body, and impaired brain function. There are two components to iron, one of which is found in meat and fish and the other which is found in plant-based sources. You need both, so if you are a vegetarian or vegan, then you will need to take an iron supplement. If you don't eat red meat but do eat fish, shellfish and canned sardines are excellent sources of iron. Plant-based sources of iron include beans, dark leafy vegetables, and seeds.

Iodine deficiency can result in mental deficiencies in developing children, shortness of breath, and weight gain. Good sources of iodine include fish, seaweed, eggs, and dairy.

Vitamin D deficiency can be identified by symptoms including muscle weakness, loss of bone density, and reduced efficacy of the immune system. Good dietary sources of vitamin D include egg yolks, fatty fish, and cod liver oil.

Vitamin B12 is only found in small amounts in food, so it is a vitamin for which a supplement or injection may be required. Vitamin B12 levels are also impacted by chronic medication, so anyone taking such medication should get a prescription for vitamin B12 injections on a monthly basis. Symptoms of vitamin B12 deficiency include a decline in mood and cognitive function, a lack of energy, and a weakened immune system. Vitamin B12 is found in shellfish, milk products, eggs, and meat.

Calcium deficiency is especially concerning in children and also as we age as it plays a major role in the formation and strength of bones. In older people, a lack of calcium may result in osteoporosis. Calcium is a mineral that is not well-absorbed from supplements, and we are far better off getting our intake from dietary sources. Foods that are high in calcium include dark green vegetables, dairy products, and boned fish.

Vitamin A deficiency is the world's leading cause of blindness, especially in developing countries where diets may not be well-rounded. This is uncommon in Western diet. A normal, well-rounded diet for a person in the United States, for instance, contains more than enough vitamin A to avoid deficiency. Dietary sources of vitamin A include sweet potatoes, fish liver oil, carrots (they really are good for the eyes!), and dark-green, leafy vegetables.

Magnesium deficiency can result in type 2 diabetes, metabolic syndrome, heart disease, and osteoporosis. Some of the symptoms of magnesium deficiency include muscle cramps, restless leg syndrome, fatigue, migraines, and abnormal heart rhythm. Magnesium is found in high levels in nuts, dark chocolate, whole grains, and dark-green, leafy vegetables.

Hyponatremia

This condition occurs when you lose salt and water through perspiration and only replace it with water. Although large amounts of salt are not good for us, sodium is actually an essential electrolyte in the body. It serves to maintain the balance of fluid around the cells which ensures proper muscle and nerve function. Sodium levels in the blood also directly correlate with blood pressure levels. When hyponatremia sets in, the concentration of sodium in your blood drops, and you may struggle to think clearly and develop headaches. This will not occur from normal day-to-day perspiration, but it may occur if you exercise while fasting or if you live in an extremely hot climate and spend a lot of time outdoors. If you are fasting and perspiring significantly as well, you can try to avoid hyponatremia by placing a pinch of salt on your tongue or adding it to a glass of water.

Orthostatic Hypotension

Hypotension is the medical term for low blood pressure, and it can be a very common occurrence during fasting. Orthostatic hypotension is a sudden decrease in blood pressure which occurs when you stand up or switch position quickly. The physical symptoms of hypotension include lightheadedness and dizziness. Hypotension can result from too much water intake, so it is important to find your personal requirement of water and stick to that. Hypotension during fasting is one of the reasons that it is so important to ensure that you are able to rest and not carry out any strenuous activities while fasting. If orthostatic hypotension becomes so bad that you cannot move at all without experiencing severe dizziness, it is best to end your fast. This condition can be avoided by good preparation as it is often a side effect of poor nutrition in the run-up to the fast or an excessive amount of toxins being expelled from the system.

Worsening of Diabetes Symptoms

Although fasting has been known to aid in the reduction of symptoms in many diabetes sufferers, it can also have the opposite effect in some individuals. Anyone with type 1 or type 2 diabetes should be very careful when considering water fasting and always consult their doctor before doing so.

It may be pertinent at this point to explain the difference between type 1 and type 2 diabetes so that the impact of water fasting and adjusting glucose levels can be fully understood. Diabetes mellitus, which we refer to colloquially as diabetes, is a disease of the metabolic system which results in blood sugar rising to dangerously high levels. Insulin is a hormone that helps to convert sugar into energy that is stored in our cells. When someone has diabetes, their body has one of two reactions to insulin. It either can't produce enough insulin, or it doesn't recognize insulin as what it is and can't effectively use it. When high blood sugar is left untreated or remains sustained for long periods of time even with treatment, the eyes, nerves, kidneys, and many other organs in the body can be affected and damaged.

Type 2 diabetes is probably the most common form and the form that we associate, quite rightly, with controllable causes. Type 2 occurs when your body becomes resistant to the insulin it produces, and therefore, it does not break down the sugar in your blood. The sugar levels then build up, and additional insulin must be introduced in order to reduce these levels.

Type 1 diabetes is actually an autoimmune disease and is far less controllable in terms of risk factors than type 2 diabetes. Type 1 diabetes develops when your immune system starts to see the pancreatic cells as pathogens rather than as a part of your body. These cells are responsible for producing insulin, so when the immune system continuously attacks them, they cannot do their job.

Other forms of diabetes include prediabetes, which is a consistent elevation of blood sugar but is not severe enough for a diagnosis of type 2 diabetes. In patients with prediabetes, fasting is an excellent method of treatment as weight loss is usually the first point of call for reducing the risk of developing full-blown type 2 diabetes. Another form of diabetes is called gestational diabetes and occurs, as the name suggests, only during pregnancy (Watson, 2020).

While the risk remains that water fasting may worsen the symptoms of already diagnosed type 2 diabetes, it is important to remember that water fasting can also be a powerful preventative measure in developing diabetes in the first place. If you are at high risk for developing diabetes—family history of diabetes, overweight or obese, and living a sedentary lifestyle—then a study conducted in June 2014 shows that a water fast for one day per week can help to reduce these risk factors significantly (Gunnars, 2019).

Another condition that may be affected negatively by fasting is gout. Gout is a complex form of arthritis which affects joints in sudden attacks. The treatment for gout involves maintaining low levels of uric acid. Fasting may, therefore, also worsen the symptoms of gout as water fasting leads to increased uric acid production, which is a known risk factor for attacks of gout.

Worsening of Eating Disorders

As most eating disorders develop around a psychological link between control and food, the act of voluntarily abstaining from food during a fast may trigger such disorders. Anyone who is living with an eating disorder or who has suffered from one in the past should carefully consider whether water fasting is the healthiest option for them both physically and emotionally. Eating disorders such as anorexia nervosa are extremely common in young females, and it is for this reason that fasting is not recommended in people under the age of 18, and it should be undertaken with great care in very young adults. Anyone that is already underweight or very close to underweight should never attempt fasting as it is very easy to slip under the ideal weight range simply through water weight loss. The most distinct line between an eating disorder and fasting is that an eating disorder is obsessive whereas fasting is intended to clear out the mind and body of any negative habits or obsessions. If at any time during fasting you feel that you may be developing a psychological obsession with the practice, you should stop immediately and seek medical guidance. While fasting can be a great weight loss tool, it should never be used compulsively for this reason.

WHO SHOULD NOT PRACTICE WATER FASTING

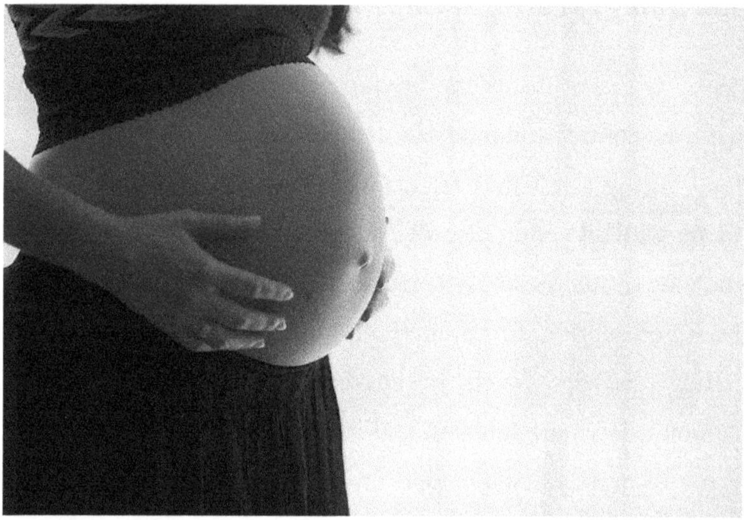

There are a few individual situations in which water fasting is not recommended. These include:

- Women who are trying to conceive or are already pregnant or breastfeeding. Women in these stages of their lives need a high level of nutrition, and the body needs to be able to focus its energy on the reproduction and gestation functions.
- Anyone under the age of 18. Children are still growing, and their bodies are developing, which necessitates a far greater need for nutrition that adults.

If you want to assist a child with better health, focus on feeding them a healthy diet and increasing their physical activity.

- Anyone who is underweight. If you suspect that you may be underweight, have this confirmed by a medical professional and undertake an eating plan that is specially developed to help you gain weight.
- Anyone with a history of eating disorders or who is currently living with an eating disorder. The restriction of food in fasting can trigger disorders that revolve around an obsession with the control of eating.
- People living with cardiovascular disorders. While fasting is good for preventing cardiovascular disorders, the sudden shifts in blood pressure and heart rate which can occur during fasting can be dangerous. Such people may also be taking chronic medication which needs to be taken with food in order to be absorbed properly.
- People living with type 1 diabetes. Those with type 2 diabetes should exercise caution when water fasting. Both of these forms of diabetes can be worsened by fasting. While significant evidence exists for its aid in relieving symptoms, the risk exists that it may have the opposite effect.
- People who regularly suffer with debilitating migraines. Headaches can be a side effect of fasting as

part of the detoxification process, and if you regularly suffer with intense migraines, this may trigger such an episode. The medication required to ease a migraine also needs to be taken with food. If you suffer from migraines and would like to try fasting, it is preferable to first seek the cause of the migraines, eliminate them as far as possible, and then try fasting.

- Anyone who has recently undergone a blood transfusion or who may have a surgery coming up that may involve a blood transfusion. This also applies to people who have recently received organ transplants. As autophagy affects the cells in your body, this may have a negative impact on someone who has received a transfusion or transplant as the immune system is impacted and may cause rejection.
- Anyone on chronic medication should consult their doctor before practicing water fasting as it is possible for certain medications to react poorly to fasting conditions in the body.
- Anyone with chronic kidney disease. When you fast, your body works very hard to remove toxins from the body. The kidneys are our main toxin-removal system, and if they are already impaired, fasting will put far too much pressure on them.

There are also circumstances which should be dealt with before water fasting is commenced. This could include periods of intense emotional stress such as grieving a death, divorce, starting a new job, or moving house. In order to be successful with water fasting, you will need to focus your mental energies on sticking to the practice, so it makes things more difficult for you if you start when you are already under severe pressure. In such an instance, wait until you have been able to move past these circumstances and then focus all of your attention on water fasting from the start.

Those who work in intense environments where focus is literally a matter of life and death, such paramedics, firefighters, police officers, and emergency room doctors, should consider starting water fasting when they are on vacation in order to avoid any loss of focus at work.

While it is nice to have family and friends who support your fasting journey, it is not absolutely necessary. You can choose whether you decide to tell people outside of your immediate family that you are fasting, but, often, doing so can just add more pressure on you. Immediate family members will likely be impacted by your fast, so while you may need to tell them that you plan on fasting, you don't need their approval. At the very least, they should just commit to not making your fast more difficult for you. Generally, you will know which people in your life are most often supportive of your choices and which are not. This is a good guideline to use in selecting who you will tell about your journey.

IS WATER FASTING SAFE?

Except for the rare few situations in which individuals should be cautious, water fasting is safe. The most important factor to consider is your individual response to the practice. Listen to your body and work within your personal health boundaries in order to achieve the best results for your situation. You know how your body reacts in certain situations, and you are the best judge of whether water fasting is the right practice for you or not. As a beginner faster, it is really not recommended that you launch into a three-day-long fast on your first try. You will still get benefits from fasting for shorter periods, so there is really no need, and it is also not advisable to push yourself too far. That said, some people would prefer to do just two longer fasts per year, for instance, rather than many shorter water fasts throughout the year. How long and how often you water fast for is going to depend completely on your personal lifestyle and what works for you. You will likely go into fasting with a preconceived idea of how you may react and what the experience will be like, and you will also likely come out the other end with a very different picture. Approach your water fast as an adventure. Adventures are exciting and interesting, but even on the most exciting of journeys, you always apply common sense and keep yourself safe—water fasting is no different. Water fasting safety should start from the minute you consider it as an option. Choose your resources wisely, consume the information you are supplied with critically and with an enquiring state of mind, and always ensure you focus on postfast behavior, including safely breaking a fast. We will delve into greater detail on the correct way to break a fast in future chapters.

3

SCIENCE-BACKED HEALTH BENEFITS OF WATER FASTING

Before we delve into guidelines for water fasting, it is imperative for me to present to you the scientific basis for the benefits that water fasting brings. This should not only give you peace of mind but also help you to understand exactly what is happening in your body when you are fasting. By understanding the mechanics of how water fasting impacts your body and how it produces the results that it does, you can also develop a realistic expectation of what you wish to achieve from water fasting. You should never attempt any health regimen or practice without fully understanding how it impacts your body. It is easy for any self-professed expert to feed you information that may seem logical. You have to live with your body for the rest of your life, though, and along with that, any damage that may be caused by following poor advice. Always ensure that you take responsibility for acquiring the knowledge you need to make wise decisions, and once you have acquired that knowledge, follow it to the tee to ensure that you are practicing fasting (or any other regimen) safely. Hype and empty promises are a dime a dozen, and anyone that would like to sell you their idea can sound convincing. Science is king, though. Empirical, fact-based data is the only way to ascertain whether a regimen is really what it purports to be. Thankfully, fasting has such research and data to back up the claims of benefits that it makes.

ACTIVATION OF AUTOPHAGY

The word autophagy literally translates to "self-eating." Thankfully, there is no cannibalism involved here, though, and the process goes on within our bodies without us even knowing it is happening. The process of autophagy involves the body breaking down and destroying old, damaged, or diseased cells and then recycling that cellular material into new, healthy cells. The process is almost constant and highly accelerated when we are young, but as we begin to age, autophagy naturally slows down. This slowing down of the autophagy process is essentially what leads to aging in humans, and the build of diseased and damaged cells contributes to diseases such as cancer, Alzheimer's disease, and other degenerative diseases. This concept is called autointoxication. Autointoxication happens when the body is negatively impacted by a toxin that it produces itself as a by-product of normal cellular function. Until relatively recently, we didn't understand how fasting regimens, including water fasting, actually caused the body to promote longevity and avoid illness, but we have now discovered the link between fasting and autophagy, which makes it clear. Autophagy, being a natural process, had for a long time been thought to be out of our control in terms of activation and acceleration. It is now clear, however, that the conditions produced when the body is in a fasted state trigger the autophagy process. As autophagy occurs in all cells in the body, this explains the overall impact of fasting on health including greater cognitive functioning as the diseased and damaged cells in the brain are consumed and replaced with healthier, younger cells. When we fast, instead of digesting food, our body can focus on digesting the toxins and waste cellular matter that are not beneficial to our health. This process of detoxification will start with the most recently acquired or developed toxins and then move on to the older toxins. Therefore, the longer you are able to fast, the more headway will be made in detoxifying your body.

Water fasting can also be very beneficial in the run up to a surgical procedure. When you activate autophagy, you will increase your rate of healing and, therefore, decrease the time it takes to heal from an operation or other procedure. The length of fast in such a case must be balanced with the point at which the procedure is set to take place. While we are ordinarily asked to fast the day before a medical procedure, this is to ensure that the anesthesia works effectively. It would not be viable or safe to end a three-day fast right before you need to go in for surgery. Preferably the fast should be completed at least a week before so that your body has time to recover from the fast slowly and correctly and that you also have time to start taking in good nutrition before you go in for your operation. Once you have been operated on and you are no longer taking heavy pain medication, where applicable, you can also embark on another fast to increase your rate of healing postoperatively. All of this should be discussed with a doctor or your proposed surgeon before the surgery.

Studies

A study conducted and published in August 2010 sought to establish the efficacy of autophagy in regenerating new and healthy brain cells. While it had been well-established in past clinical studies that autophagy cleaned up cells in many areas of the body, at this time, the medical community was uncertain about the real impact on brain cells. All clinical studies start with animal subjects as it does not require special clearance, and such studies are far less complicated than those with human participants. Basic anatomy is very similar in all mammals, though, so results gleaned from animal subjects can easily be extrapolated to human results. Researchers in this study food-restricted rodent subjects for 24 to 48 hours in order to see the impact that fasting, and as a result, autophagy, had on the subjects' brain cells. The results indicated that brain cells showed as much improvement in condition from fasting as the cells in other areas of the body (Alirezaei et al., 2010).

The link between fasting, autophagy, and possible increased longevity was explored in another study conducted in 2015. The thinking behind the link is that if we are able to replace old, damaged cells which lead to aging on a more consistent basis, then we should be able to increase the lifespan of those cells, and as a whole, the body. The connection between the build-up of damaged and diseased cells and chronic illness is also another idea behind this theory. In this study, middle-aged rodent subjects were subjected to a diet which mimics fasting in the body, and the long-term results of this were measured by comparing the postfast levels of hormones and organic compounds which are linked to longevity. In these subjects, it was found that the fasting conditions helped to extend longevity, lowered body fat levels, reduced the incidence of cancer in subjects, and improved immune system functioning (Brandhorst et al., 2015).

A third study published in 2008 investigated the link between fasting, autophagy, and a decrease in markers for chronic disease. The research determined that there is significant evidence to conclude that autophagy can help to defend against metabolic stress. It works as a housekeeper at a cellular level by cleaning out all of the unnecessary parts, reducing the build-up of cellular material in the brain which leads to degenerative brain disease, has a similar effect in degenerative muscles diseases, and can help prevent cancer (Levine & Kroemer), 2008).

AIDS IN WEIGHT LOSS

One of the main reasons that fasting has become so popular is because of its ability to aid weight loss. When done properly, weight that is lost through water fasting is not regained as is the case with many fad fasts. In order to set realistic goals for ourselves and have measured expectations, it is important to understand exactly how fasting impacts the body in order to result in weight loss.

One of the predominant ways that water fasting helps to aid in weight loss is by boosting your metabolism. When we are in a fasted state, the levels of norepinephrine in our body increase. This neurotransmitter plays a key role in boosting our metabolism.

The point that we need to get to in order to lose weight is fat burning. Fat burning for energy only happens after the glucose energy stores in our body are depleted. When we maintain a fed state, we don't give our body a chance to get to the fat stores, as it is constantly using the food that you are giving it in the form of glucose stores in order to fuel the body's processes. When you fast, though, you are giving your body the opportunity to use up the glucose stores and then move on to burning the fat stores. The rate at which fasting aids in fat burning, of course, depends on how many glucose and fat stores you have. While exercise aids the acceleration of fat burning as you are burning through energy stores more quickly than when you are in a resting state, the key to water fasting is to increase the fat burning that happens when you are in that resting state. There are domino effects to maintaining a healthy weight which go beyond self-image and appearance. Most chronic illnesses have risk factors which include obesity, including cardiovascular disease and type 2 diabetes. Doctors from the University of Oxford in the United Kingdom also explain that besides weight loss, the burning of fat for energy results in the preservation of muscle and the reduction of cholesterol levels (Gunnars, 2019).

The Academy of Nutrition and Dietetics notes that the most efficient way to lose weight and ensure it is kept off is to follow the process slowly, eat a healthy diet, and increase physical activity (Gunnars, 2019). This, of course, is sometimes easier said than done, and the struggle to lose weight becomes an ongoing, lifelong journey. One of the biggest issues with losing weight is our relationship with food. Many have developed an emotional connection to eating, and as such, we eat when we are happy, sad, or experiencing any emotion in between. It is also this emotional connection with food that leads to food addictions such as sugar, caffeine, junk food, and overeating. All of these emotional connections have a negative outcome as we begin to gain weight, become diseased, and generally feel unwell. The irony often is that the more weight we gain, the worse we feel about ourselves and the more we eat. This, of course, only leads to further weight gain and a vicious circle ensues. Water fasting can help us to reset our relationship with food. In later chapters, I will discuss the importance of prefast preparation. If you have a particularly emotional relationship with food, you will want to allocate a longer period to your prefast preparations as you are going to be using this time to start reducing your food addictions and emotional bonds to food. During your water fast, you should spend as much time as possible reflecting on how these addictions and emotional connections formed. It is not uncommon for obesity to be rooted in emotional trauma, and this is why anyone who advocates fasting understands that it is a mind and body experience. Be prepared for some issues to be raised while you are fasting that you may not have been consciously aware of, and if appropriate, seek counseling to help you move past these issues. By treating your emotional and mental health, you can significantly impact your body. This will also set you on a path to greater success in weight loss through fasting.

In order to set realistic weight loss goals, we need to consider that we did not gain the weight that we now wish to lose overnight. We will, therefore, also not lose the weight overnight. From a mental health perspective, it is important for us to set realistic goals. When we set outrageous goals for weight loss, we set ourselves up for failure and not only do we not lose any weight but we also lose hope. The best way of setting weight loss goals is by breaking them down into smaller achievable chunks that you can easily measure and setting time periods for those achievements. As you achieve the smaller goals, you can increase the magnitude of your goals and work your way up. I would recommend not setting any weight loss goal for your first round of water fasting. That initial experience is to get your body used to the practice and set yourself up for future, longer fasts. You can certainly use any weight that you may lose as a gauge for future fasts, but this should be done in the spirit of curiosity and do not be disappointed if you gain it back.

The fact that a lot of weight loss from initial fasting is related to water weight means that you are better off measuring your progress by using a tape measure to take your body measurements rather than using the scale. The scale doesn't know if it's weighing water, fat, or muscle, so it really does not give you an accurate understanding of how much fat you have lost—which is, of course, the ultimate weight loss goal.

Studies

In 2000, a study was published which sought to determine whether short-term fasting could result in the acceleration of energy burning in a resting state. The subjects of the study were exposed to a fasting state for various periods over an 84-hour period. Their levels of certain hormones, which represent fat burning, were measured on each of the days, and they showed a definite increase in the rate of fat burning in a short-term fast. It is believed, however, that if one stays without food for a long period, a week at a time for instance, fat burning levels will actually slow down (Zauner et al., 2000). The key, therefore, is to fast for just long enough to burn fat but not so long that you start to slow that acceleration or, indeed, do any damage to your body.

In 2015, researchers looked into the real impact of fasting on the body's composition. They measured body weight, cholesterol, body fat percentage, and triglyceride levels. The latter is an indicator, at a high level, for cardiovascular disease. The study looked at the impact of alternate-day fasting as well as whole-day fasting and found that in all cases, the levels of the aforementioned measurement criteria improved dramatically. Interestingly most measurement criteria did not increase significantly more on whole-day fasting than they did on alternate-day fasting (Tinsley, 2015).

REDUCES INFLAMMATION

Chronic inflammation in the body is another precursor for many chronic illnesses. Chronic inflammation can be caused by many factors including misdirected immune responses. The process of inflammation is actually the body's natural process to fight infection. It is a vital part of our immune system. It is only when that process starts to malfunction that inflammation becomes a problem. Inflammation occurs when the body sends a large number of white blood cells to the site of an injury or infection, but sometimes the body can mistake its own cells for pathogens, and this is the root cause of autoimmune diseases. When we are sick or injured, we experience acute inflammation. Depending on the illness or injury, this inflammation can present in different ways, or you may not experience any symptoms of the inflammation at all. When the body no longer exhibits a reduction response to the inflammation, and it continues on for many months or years, this is termed chronic inflammation. Chronic inflammation can also be caused by eating too much animal protein, living a generally unhealthy lifestyle, and not getting enough sleep.

Chronic inflammation results in a very high level of monocytes in the blood. Monocytes are proinflammation cells, and although they are necessary for activating normal inflammation, when they occur in excessive levels they become problematic. Researchers have discovered, though, that these cells seem to be more active when the body is in a fed state and less active when they are in a fasted state. In the latter state, in fact, they are almost in sleep mode and not producing any inflammatory effects at all. Dr. Stefan Jordan of the Icahn School of Medicine at Mount Sinai says that this discovery holds many positive implications for the reduction of many chronic disease levels (Staff, 2019). Fasting has specifically been shown to be beneficial in reducing the symptoms of multiple sclerosis, which is a condition characterized by chronic inflammation in the body.

Another indicator of chronic inflammation is increased levels of C-Reactive Protein (CRP) and cytokines, which are produced by the liver and immune system in response to inflammation in the body. After three days of regular water fasting, the levels of these indicators start to drop in the body.

Studies

In 2012, a study was undertaken to investigate the links between inflammation and several chronic diseases and by doing so, establish new possible treatments and preventative measures to limit the occurrence of such chronic illnesses. The study focused on prior research undertaken by various members of the medical research community. Research has found that patients with cancer have high levels of inflammation-related markers as well. In a study at the University of Washington, patients with tumors were monitored, and at each stage of tumor growth, inflammation markers were also measured. A direct correlation was found in the increase in inflammation markers and the growth of the tumor (Hunter, 2012). Diseases which relate to degeneration of the nervous system have also been linked to chronic inflammation. Such diseases include amyotrophic lateral sclerosis (ALS) which is relatively common and currently fatal in almost all cases.

Considering the distinct link between chronic inflammation and the occurrence of so many of these diseases, researchers started to look into how the prevention of chronic inflammation could be implemented. The use of traditional remedies and foods that have anti-inflammatory properties is an important area for researchers as these are methods that can be practiced throughout life and incorporated into the diet. A component of turmeric has been shown to provide significant anti-inflammatory properties, for instance.

Researchers also found significant evidence that fasting as well as exercise has a significant impact on reducing inflammation in the body (Hunter, 2012).

IMPROVES SENSITIVITY TO VARIOUS HORMONES

Fasting has been shown to improve sensitivity to hormones such as insulin and leptin. Insulin is produced by your pancreas and is used to regulate your blood sugar level and the nutrients that are transported by your bloodstream, and it impacts fat and protein metabolism. An intake of carbohydrates will signal your body to release additional insulin so that it can convert that food into glucose stores. In some people, the cells of the body will fail to correctly respond to the presence of insulin, and this can lead to a wide variety of issues including type 2 diabetes and other insulin resistance complications (Gunnars, 2019). Studies have shown that water fasting helps to reduce insulin resistance, thereby maintaining a steady blood sugar. The intake of any food increases insulin levels. It is possible to control insulin levels by taking in only certain types of foods that have a lower impact on insulin than others. This method, however, will prevent extremely high levels, but it will not do anything to decrease levels effectively. The key to preventing the body becoming resistant to insulin is to bring levels of insulin down to extremely low levels for periods at a time. The best way to achieve this is to fast.

Leptin is the hormone that your body releases in order to indicate to your brain that you are full and that you should stop eating. Just like any other hormone, it is possible to become resistant to leptin, and this is now believed to be one of the greatest contributors to weight gain. Leptin is produced by the fat cells in your body, and it works on the hypothalamus in the brain to indicate that you are full and no longer require food. This is a side-role for the hormone, though, and its main function is to regulate energy as well as the number of calories you take in and the number of fat stores available to you. The evolution of leptin was intended to avoid us starving or overeating, and while it has worked extremely well on the starvation end, modern man has seemingly hacked the overeating end, and we no longer respond to leptin's instructions in the way we should. As leptin is produced in fat cells, it stands to reason that the more fat cells you have, the more leptin you produce. When your body fat increases and your leptin levels increase too, we are supposed to eat less and burn more fat. In obese people, though, their leptin levels have become so high that their brain has become resistant to its signals. When your brain doesn't pick up the leptin signals, it believes that you are starving and will encourage you to eat more and expend less energy. By using water fasting to increase your body's sensitivity to leptin, you can avoid overeating and more easily control the feeling of hunger. This, in turn, helps to avoid becoming overweight or obese.

Studies

In a study published in 2005, researchers subjected rodent subjects to a 24-hour period of normal eating, measured their insulin and leptin levels, and then subjected them to a 48-hour fast, after which they retested their hormone levels. The subjects ranged in age from what would be considered young to what would be considered elderly in terms of rodent lifespan. Researchers found that in the initial normal feeding period, the older rats showed a lower sensitivity to insulin and leptin while the younger rats demonstrated normal levels of sensitivity. After the fasting period, all rats had the same (i.e., normal) level of sensitivity (Kmiec et al., 2005).

In another study, this time published in 2003, researchers sought to determine the impact of this hormone stabilization on brain cell degeneration. Through a mixed study which involved placing rodent subjects under fasting conditions, researchers were able to determine that the group that was fasted and showed increased sensitivity to hormones such as insulin and leptin, also showed less neural degeneration and had an overall longer lifespan than those who were allowed to eat as they pleased (Anson et al., 2003).

IMPROVES HEART HEALTH

Cardiovascular disease is one of the leading causes of death worldwide. There are several predominant risk factors to cardiovascular disease including hypertension (high blood pressure) and obesity (especially belly fat), and levels of cholesterol and triglycerides in the blood. Fasting helps to decrease the levels of these risk factors in the body and when paired with a healthy diet and improved physical activity is an excellent way to decrease the likelihood of cardiovascular diseases.

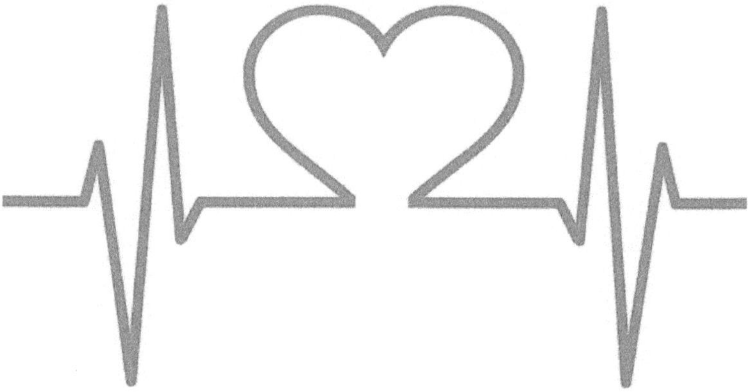

There are two types of cholesterol that exist in the body, but they are not both risk factors for heart disease. Low-density lipoprotein or LDL cholesterol is the type that we want to limit. It is known as "bad" cholesterol as it is the main source of clogged arteries. The other type of cholesterol is high-density lipoprotein or HDL. This form of cholesterol actually helps to reduce the levels of LDL in the system.

Cardiovascular disease is often diagnosed in older women, especially women who are menopausal or postmenopausal. A correlating factor to this rate of diagnosis is that belly fat is known to be far more common in women of this age range. The reason that belly fat, specifically, is so dangerous is that it is an active fat, which releases triglycerides into the blood at a far higher rate than fat in other parts of the body. Fasting is well known for its efficacy in decreasing belly fat. The presence of belly fat is one of five risk factors, which when grouped together, are referred to as metabolic syndrome. Those living with metabolic syndrome are at far higher risk of developing cardiovascular disease, diabetes, and strokes. Besides the presence of belly fat, the other four risk factors are elevated blood pressure (hypertension), high blood sugar levels, high levels of triglycerides in the blood, and low levels of good cholesterol (HDL). If you have three or more of these risk factors, you will be diagnosed with metabolic syndrome, and you will need to take urgent and consistent action to reduce the existence of these factors. Rather than waiting for too many of these risk factors to develop and a diagnosis of metabolic syndrome to emerge, it is far better to take preventative action to avoid the symptoms developing in the first place.

Free radicals can play a major role in damaging our heart as well as other parts of our body. These unstable molecules are known to cause what is called oxidative damage to parts of cells. There are foods that contain high levels of antioxidants, and these are highly beneficial, when paired with fasting, in reducing damage to the heart muscle. Examples of food that contain high levels of antioxidants include dark chocolate, pecan nuts, blueberries, artichokes, strawberries, raspberries, kale, and goji berries.

Hypertension or high blood pressure is one of the leading contributing factors to cardiovascular disease.

Studies

In a study conducted with a group of 68 people, all of whom suffered with high blood pressure issues, the participants were subjected to a fast for almost 14 days while under constant medical supervision. At the end of the period, 82% of the participants had reduced their blood pressure to normal levels (Gunnars, 2019)

In one study, 30 participants who presented as healthy adults were subjected to a water fast for just 24 hours. Their levels of cholesterol and triglycerides were measured before and after the 24-hour water fast, and it was found that their postfast levels were significantly reduced (Raman, 2019).

In another study, 174 participants suffering from hypertension were subjected to water fasting for 10 days, again under medical supervision. At the end of the 10-day period, 90% of the participants had seen a drop in blood pressure to readings that are considered normal (Raman, 2019).

In 2007, a study was undertaken to determine the impact of fasting on blood pressure, cholesterol, and triglycerides in the blood. Researchers used a group of 110 patients with a mix of male and female patients, all of whom presented with obesity. The patients were hospitalized for the duration of the study and were subjected to fasting conditions. Their blood pressure, cholesterol, and triglyceride levels were monitored before, during, and after the fasting was complete. At the end of the three-week period, all subjects had lost up to 40 pounds each. Their blood pressure levels had dropped to a normal reading, and their cholesterol and triglyceride levels had all decreased significantly (Beleslin et al., 2007).

PREVENTION OF DEGENERATIVE DISEASES AND COGNITIVE DECLINE

The degenerative diseases which are often linked with age such as Alzheimer's Disease are often seen as almost an inevitable part of ageing. The truth, though, is that scientific research is discovering that it is entirely possible to take preventative measures throughout our lives in order to significantly reduce the possibility that we will present with these diseases in old age. The basis of this idea is the link between the build-up of damaged and diseased cells and degenerative disease as well as general cognitive decline. The reason this build-up happens is because of the naturally slowing rate of autophagy in the body as we age. The body is less capable of removing damaged and diseased cells from all areas of the body, including the brain, and this build-up plays a role in cognitive decline and disease.

As we know, fasting is a trigger for autophagy, and this is the reason that we now see fasting as a preventative measure in avoiding cognitive decline and disease. Although this benefit may only seem apparent in later years, it is widely recognized that fasting boosts cognitive functioning in people of all ages. It is particularly beneficial for women who are experiencing brain fogging due to hormonal changes such as after pregnancy and during menopause. Women who have given birth should always wait until they have stopped breastfeeding to start fasting.

The link between our cognitive functioning and food, or the absence thereof, becomes clear if we consider what our own cognitive functioning is like around food. When you eat a large meal, you start to feel tired and incapable of performing cognitively. Often, you will need to go and have a nap in order to feel better. This is because, when you overload your stomach with food, your body automatically shifts the majority of blood flow to the digestive system in order to aid digestion. As a result, your brain is left to function on minimal blood flow, which is generally just enough to keep messages flowing to your muscles and organs. You feel the need to sit still or lie down as a result of your body wanting to direct that blood flow elsewhere. By the same token, when you don't eat, you feel mentally sharper. You may become hyperaware and find it easier to focus. This is physical proof of our brain's relationship with food.

There is a wide range of diseases which are considered to be degenerative in nature. These include:

- Alzheimer's disease
- Cancers

- Amyotrophic lateral sclerosis (ALs), also known as Lou Gehrig's disease
- Charcot-Marie-Tooth (CMT) disease
- Cystic fibrosis
- Chronic traumatic encephalopathy
- Huntington's disease
- Frontotemporal dementia
- Macular degeneration
- Parkinson's disease
- Rheumatoid arthritis
- Motor neuron disease

A disease is considered degenerative if it results from a consistent degradation of cells in the body which impact the functioning of organs or tissue. Once a degenerative disease has manifested, it can, in most cases be treated in terms of the symptoms, but degeneration will continue and there are no cures for most of these diseases. Many will have fatal results. The need for preventative measures cannot be overstated, especially if you already have risk factors for these diseases. If you are genetically predisposed or your lifestyle habits make you more likely to develop one of these degenerative diseases, it is imperative that you act beforehand and give your body the best chances of fighting off such a disease.

Studies

In 2013, a study was published which delved into the impact of fasting on cognitive development and functioning. The study was conducted over 11 months and started with young rodent subjects in order to track their brain development and cognitive functioning levels when exposed to different diets. One group was submitted to a constant intermittent fasting diet while the other was fed on a high fat diet. The subjects' cognitive abilities were tested throughout the study period, and by the end of the study, it was determined that the group that had been subjected to the fasting diet had far better cognitive and problem-solving abilities than the group that had been subject to the high-fat diet. There was no difference in the way the brain developed in terms of structure, but there was significant difference in the way the rodents were able to think and solve problems (Li et al., 2013).

Another study conducted in 2000 sought to determine whether the generation of new brain cells could be impacted by restricting the intake of food—in other words, fasting. Adult rodent subjects were put into a fasted state for intermittent periods of time during the study. The levels of new brain cell generation as well as the release of Brain Derived Neurotrophic Factor (BDNF) were measured. BDNF is a hormone that when present in higher levels is known to increase the rate of neural cell generation. All subjects showed increased levels of all tested criteria after fasting (Lee et al., 2000).

INCREASED SECRETION OF HUMAN GROWTH HORMONE

Human Growth Hormone (HGH) is a hormone produced by your pituitary gland that plays a key role in the body. It is involved in growth, weight loss, metabolism, and muscle strength. Levels of HGH decrease in the body as we age, and this is one of the reasons that older people find it more difficult to lose weight and experience muscle wastage and loss of strength. Your diet and lifestyle can impact the levels of HGH in your body at any age.

Research has shown that water fasting could help to increase HGH levels in the body, regardless of age. The ability of water fasting to help maintain steady blood sugar and insulin levels also helps to increase levels of the hormone, as consistently peaked insulin levels have been shown to reduce HGH in the blood.

HGH is also increased further by losing body fat, and there is a direct correlation between the amount of belly fat in the body and the levels of HGH. The more belly fat that a person has, the lower their levels of HGH. Arginine is a supplement that can be taken while water fasting that helps to increase HGH levels as well. If you are specifically looking to increase your HGH levels while water fasting, use your preparation time to cut out all of your sugar intake. When sugar levels are high, so is insulin and as a result HGH is suppressed. The time at which you eat when you have broken your fast also makes a difference in your HGH levels. Eating too close to bedtime is not only bad for your digestive system, but it reduces your HGH levels.

Studies

In 2012, researchers were able to determine that during a 24-hour fast, levels of HGH increased in study participants. Another study also showed that levels of HGH increased by five times the nonfasted level, in participants who were subjected to a 24 to 48-hour fast (Salgin, 2012).

In one study conducted over one week of fasting, researchers found that within three days of fasting, participants' HGH levels had increased by 300%. After a full week of fasting, these levels had increased by 1,250%. Other studies indicated a tripling of HGH levels after just two days of fasting (Salgin, 2012).

APPLIED BENEFITS

The benefits of water fasting and autophagy can be applied in several areas to improve health. Researchers are now looking at using fasting as a complementary treatment for cancer patients who are on chemotherapy as it helps to improve the removal of dead and diseased cells and replace them with healthy cells that are more likely to fight the disease. Fasting may also make chemotherapy more effective in the body while reducing the side effects of the treatment. A study conducted on the growth of tumor cells showed that cyclical fasting was as effective as chemotherapy in retarding the growth of tumor cells. Medical advice should always be sought before commencing fasting as a complementary treatment while taking chemotherapy.

Water fasting can also be beneficial in many autoimmune diseases as it helps to reboot the immune system and may reduce the symptoms of several autoimmune diseases such as inflammation. When you incur an injury or suffer from a disease, your body sends white blood cells to the site in question to aid in healing. White blood cells, just like other cells of the body, have a limited lifespan, and as they age, they become less effective. Stem cells are those that give rise to new white blood cells, and it has been shown that water fasting activates stem cells to produce new white blood cells and rejuvenate the immune system. A significant figure in the fasting research community, Dr. Valter Longo, conducted a study with a research team from the University of Southern California to investigate the true impact of fasting on the immune system. The team found that water fasting of between two and four days in length can renew many of the cells in the immune system and effectively reboot it. Dr. Longo explains that when you do not take calories in, your body saves energy by recycling many of the cells of the immune system that are not required as well as those that may be damaged or ineffective. Longo went on to demonstrate that in people whose immune systems are already significantly damaged, such as those on chemotherapy, this process can effectively rebuild an entire immune system (Gunnars, 2019).

The process of autophagy, which replaces dead and diseased cells with new cells, will also have the applied benefit of increasing overall longevity. While this theory has only been tested and proven in animal subjects, the science behind the theory certainly indicates that the same would be applicable to humans. The fact that water fasting and autophagy definitely reduce our risk of developing several chronic diseases also contributes to the idea that lifespan would be increased by this practice.

From the perspective of appearance, wrinkling and sagging of skin occur as we age predominantly because our body produces far less collagen than it did when we were younger. Collagen is a protein in the blood that helps to provide structure to the skin and aids in the clotting of blood. Fasting has been shown to promote healthier levels of collagen in the skin, thereby improving skin structure and appearance.

Overall, fasting helps to improve our relationship with food. If you really sit and consider how much time you spend every day thinking and talking about, and preparing food, you will likely be amazed at how much of your time it takes up. When we structure our eating by water fasting, we free up our minds to focus on other areas of our lives. The modern way of eating, which basically involves being in a constantly fed state, has damaged our relationship with food. Rather than seeing food as something that nourishes our body, we have started to see it as something that we need to have constantly available to us. In some cases, this can actually lead to emotional disorders developing around food where it is used as an emotional crutch. This constantly fed state has also impacted our understanding of hunger. Most human beings today do not understand what true hunger is or what it feels like. We mistake boredom, emotional disturbance, and even thirst for hunger. By implementing water fasting as a lifestyle, we can reset our brain's understanding and response to true hunger and help our bodies to reach a more natural state in this regard.

Water fasting, in particular, has additional applied benefits to ordinary intermittent or other forms of fasting. Water, of course, is an extremely important substance to the human body. When we drink water, it is not absorbed in the same way that food is. While food is digested, water is absorbed directly into our system. This rate of absorption is far higher when our stomach is empty, though. Drinking water improves hydration levels, energy level, and physical performance. It also supports the growth of hair and the composition of skin. Water is absolutely necessary to ensure that functions in the body, including brain function, continue correctly. This is one of the reasons that when you start to become dehydrated, you also develop a brain fog. Severe dehydration can even lead to hallucinations as your brain functions start to completely shut down. Several forms of headaches and migraines can actually be caused by not having sufficient hydration levels, which is why doctors recommend drinking a large glass of water before taking any pain medication for a headache. After waiting about half an hour, you will be able to see whether there is any easing of pain, and if so, you will know that your headache was actually caused by dehydration. When we fast and increase the autophagy process, we produce more waste material that needs to be removed. Our kidneys are the predominant organ involved in flushing toxins from our bodies. In order for our kidneys to work efficiently, they need water. Sweating is another way that our body gets rid of toxins, and water is also required for this process. The more we sweat, the more we need to replace that lost fluid by drinking more water.

In comparison to other plans which simply require a restriction of calories, fasting has been found to be far more effective at reducing weight while, importantly, preserving muscle tissue. Water fasting is also a far safer way to induce ketosis (fat burning) in your body. It avoids a state called metabolic acidosis which can be common in low-carb, high-fat diets. Metabolic acidosis occurs when ketones build up in the body due to ketosis being too quickly achieved for too long a period. The kidneys struggle to remove these ketones and their resultant acid from the body and, as a result, the body slowly begins to be poisoned.

Another resultant benefit of fasting is that your body intuitively knows where to send blood, and when you are fasting, your digestive system, which usually uses the largest supply of blood, no longer needs it. As a result, increased blood flow is sent to your lungs and skin, both of which are excellent organs of detoxification.

The emotional and mental health benefits of fasting are significant and proven. When the detoxification process starts to occur and fat is burned for energy, we experience a state in our body which is similar to exercise. Endorphins or "feel good" hormones are released at this stage, and this results in an intense feeling of well-being and happiness. A reduced rate of endorphin production is one of the risk factors for mental health diseases like depression and anxiety. Mental health disorders like these affect at least 25% of the global population. The release of additional BDNF as well as the decreased levels of inflammation in the body have both been shown to aid in reducing the severity of depression. Many pharmaceutical antidepressants work to increase the level of BDNF in the body, and while it is not intended to replace antidepressants at all, fasting may definitely help in making their work easier. Another interesting link can be made between the impact that fasting has on the helpful bacteria in our gut and our mental health and brain activity. The bacteria that live in our gut are called microbiota, and they play a surprising role in our body. Microbiota are not just useful in aiding digestion; they also play a role in sending signals to the immune system to maintain its proper functioning and in turn influence levels of inflammation, which plays a role in depression. A direct link between the gut and the brain has been established, and imbalances in one have been shown to directly impact the other. The benefit of fasting in restoring gut health is, therefore, another way in which it plays a role in mental health (Rose, n.d.). Fasting should never replace psychotherapy or pharmaceutical aids in people suffering from severe depression or anxiety, but it can certainly play a role in aiding the reduction of symptoms.

4

GETTING STARTED WITH WATER FASTING

As with any new journey which aligns with specific goals, planning is imperative to ensure that you can reach your goal safely. Water fasting is no different. In order to get the best results possible out of water fasting and to practice it safely, it is important to understand the prefasting practices which should be followed. By following the preparation steps which I will lay out in this chapter, you will radically improve your chances of success.

WHAT TO CONSIDER BEFORE WATER FASTING

Setting a time period for your first water fast should be determined by your experience in fasting. If you have never fasted before, it is better to start with a shorter period and work your way up. A 24-hour period should be sufficient to start, but if even that sounds a bit too much to begin with, feel free to start on a shorter period and slowly increase. The reasons for starting small and working up are several. You will experience some side effects as your body starts to adjust to no longer being constantly fed, and by building up your fasting period, you give yourself an opportunity to slowly work through those side effects rather than experiencing them all at once. Many people who fail at water fasting try to go for too long a period on their first occasion, and when they suddenly experience many side effects at once, on top of dealing with hunger, the experience becomes overwhelming and they quit. If you had no experience with running, you wouldn't go out for a 20-mile jog on your first day, would you? You would start with a walk around the block and then a run, and then you would build up your distance bit-by-bit. The same concept applies to fasting. Water fasting may not be exercise in the true sense of the word, but just as exercise puts a form of stress on your body (good stress in this context), so does fasting. That is why it is vital to get your body used to this new way of being slowly and gradually.

If you are currently in a constantly fed state, you put yourself at risk for nutritional deficiencies by suddenly reducing your food intake. This is another reason that your run-up to the water fast is so important. A good way to start is with one 24-hour water fast per week. After a few weeks of successful 24-hour water fasts, you can start to build yourself up to a 48-hour fast. Those who are obese or suffer from chronic inflammation can try and build up their fasts to longer than three days, keeping in mind that your body needs to get used to consuming only water, and many people may not cope well with extended periods of water fasting.

Educating yourself about water fasting is one of the most important parts of preparation. By reading this book, you are doing exactly that. As I have mentioned in other parts of this book, if you are living with a chronic condition or take prescription medicine, it is important to consult a doctor before starting water fasting, just to ensure that you understand how a fasted state might interact with your medication or condition.

PICK YOUR MOMENT

Water fasting is not something that can be done on the spur of the moment due to its intensity. You will need to choose a time when you are not experiencing any major stress or changes in your life. It is also preferable to be able to spend most of your time in a rested state while you are fasting and not undertake any strenuous activities. Your body is going to be in a major period of healing and repair, and it needs to be able to focus the bulk of its energy on carrying out those internal activities.

If you are feeling physically or emotionally unwell, do not start your water fasting at that time. Use your fasting time to enrich your mind and soul. Spend time reading, enjoying the company of pets, and sleeping as much as you can. Your body heals really when you are asleep as it doesn't need to expend energy on thinking or moving muscles. A good time to start water fasting could be over a weekend or when you are on vacation and spending time at home.

If you want to do an extended fast and aren't able to take time off work, then you can attempt the fast with your normal routine, but this is not recommended for first-time fasts. You will not know how your body is going to react until you start fasting, so it really is better if you allow yourself time to adjust in a safe space.

PREPARE YOUR BODY

The changes that your body is going to undergo when you are water fasting are quite dramatic and, in order to get the most out of the fast, it is important to ensure that your body is prepared for the water fast beforehand. Think about it as preparing yourself for battle. In the days before your water fast, you will need to be really selective and purposeful about what you put into your body. Your body cannot make the changes it needs to if you have fed it junk beforehand. Also consider that one of the main processes you want to accelerate is the burning of fat, and in order to get to that stage, you need to burn through your glucose stores first. If you eat a lot of processed and refined carbohydrates in the days before your fast, your body will have a lot more glucose stores to work through before you get to the fat-burning stage. This clean and healthy eating preparation period should last at least one week before your fast (two weeks if you can manage it). An easy way to do this is simply by reducing the number of unhealthy snacks or treats you allow yourself per day and start to reduce the portion size you are consuming when you eat. You want to give your digestive system the best chance possible to perform well during a fast, so it is important to avoid difficult to digest foods such as animal proteins and dairy products in the preparation period before your water fast. Plenty of fruit and vegetables are vital for their nutrients and fiber content. Organic produce is always best as you are ensured that you are not taking in chemicals or the like, but if you are unable to get organic, as long as the produce is fresh, that is completely fine. Increase the amount of antioxidant-rich foods you take in during your preparation period to ensure that the destruction of free radicals is optimized during your fast.

During this preparation period, get into the habit of increasing your hydration and relying on water as a substitute for food. This will make it much easier for you when you start water fasting as your brain will already be accustomed to seeing water as satisfying. This is also a good time to prepare the quality of water that you plan to drink during your fast. Depending on the area you live in, you might have access to decent quality tap water. Even if it is drinkable, though, tap water rarely contains the same amount of minerals that bottled water does. Bottled water can get expensive, though, so you should consider investing in a high-quality reverse osmosis filter system for your home so that you can convert tap water to high quality water within the comfort of your own home at no cost to you. Salt as electrolytes is also an important consideration, and the quality of salt you consume also makes a huge difference. You can use this preparation time to find the best quality salt that you can afford. The best salts are ideally sea salts, and you can add some to your drinking water to get in those much-needed electrolytes.

One of the best ways to get in a lot of fresh produce and ease up on your digestive system is by drinking vegetable and fruit smoothies in the run up to your fast. Smoothies are also a great way to take in natural anti-inflammatories like turmeric. It may be a good idea to ease your body into water fasting by drinking smoothies only for a day or so before you commence your fast.

Also during this period, try to reduce anything that you may take in that could result in toxins in your body. This includes alcohol, cigarettes, refined sugary drinks, and any over-the-counter medication that you may take regularly. The intensity of the side effects you experience during water fasting will be in direct correlation to the amount of toxins you are putting into your body just before the water fast. If you live a high-toxin life-style such as smoking, drinking an excessive amount of alcohol, eating poorly, and not exercising, you can expect to experience a significant number of high-intensity side effects if you go straight from that lifestyle into water fasting. This is why I highly recommend taking a week or two before you start your first water fast to gradually change your lifestyle and allow your body to start moving those toxins out.

Some experts recommend starting with intermittent fasting in the days before your extended water fast starts as this can start to prepare your body to enter ketosis more quickly. Intermittent fasting is when you have a fasting window and an eating window within the same 24-hour period.

GET MOVING MODERATELY

Moderate exercise is a very beneficial part of your preparation for a water fast. Select activities that you look forward to doing so that you are maintaining good emotional stability. Yoga and meditation are both great for your prefast preparation as they exercise both the mind and the body and help you get into a centered and mindful place, which will be vital for a successful fast. A daily walk in the park (with a dog if you have one) has a calming effect which helps to reduce stress levels. It is important to avoid really strenuous exercise in the period before your water fast, and also while you are fasting. Ensure that you get lots of sleep and rest in this period as well.

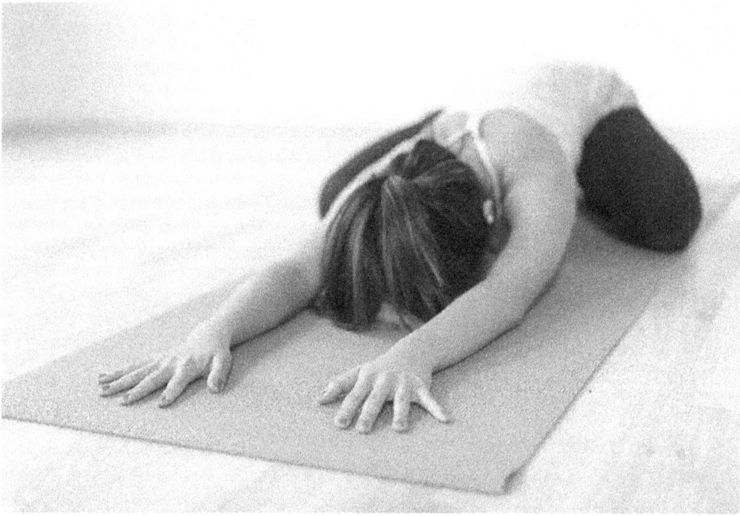

Yoga is an exercise that fits in really well with the fasting lifestyle. Its focus on mindfulness, breath exercise, and meditation is beneficial in keeping the mind focused during fasting. You don't need to go to a yoga class to enjoy yoga. There are many online classes as well as DVDs focused on teaching yoga to beginners. Meditation is a mind exercise that is really helpful in staying focused on your goals. While you may picture a monk sitting cross-legged in a temple when you think about meditation, it is really much simpler than that. The point of meditation is to clear your mind and be present in the moment. To do this you will need a quiet area. The idea behind meditation is that you don't need to push things out of your mind. As you sit and focus on your breathing, ideas, thoughts, and emotions will inevitably pop into your head. When they do, don't become frustrated with yourself; simply acknowledge the thought or emotion without judgment and allow it to move on. This concept of mindfulness is very helpful in reducing any anxiety you might feel about the water fasting process. It is almost impossible to feel any anxiety if you are in the present moment. Anxiety is about past and future events, not current events, so if you are focused only on what is happening right now, anxiety is not a concern. When you are fasting, mindfulness is a great tool to keep you grounded and centered. If you don't already practice mindfulness or meditation, try to include this in your preparation period so that you can be adept at it during your water fast.

Stretching is another great exercise during your fast. It is a low-impact exercise but really helps to improve flexibility in your muscles and get your blood flowing. Stretching will be especially beneficial if you are used to high-impact exercises under normal circumstances and you are missing that while you are fasting. By stretching twice daily, you will keep your muscles supple and reduce stiffness. Stretching is particularly good for those over 40 who may start to experience the aches and pains associated with age. Back pain is one of the most common complaints in people of that age group, and stretching can help to improve the strength of core muscles and encourages better posture, which is often the root cause of back pain. Stretching exercises are a surprisingly good stress reliever and, as with yoga, as you begin to focus on the movement of your body and your breathing, it's easier to move the stresses of the moment out of your mind. If you are struggling with headaches during your fasting, stretching may help to relieve them as well. If you are new to stretching, there is a proper form that you need to follow in order to avoid injury. There are several online resources and books that will teach you the correct way to stretch and give you an idea of what sort of stretching you should be doing. Stretching is rather more involved than the stretch you do when you get out of bed in the morning so be sure to do your homework and some research before starting.

PREPARE YOURSELF MENTALLY

It is often the unexpected side effects of a water fast that cause people to fail. If you have an unrealistic expectation of what fasting will be like, and then you are met with a very different reality, this may be the cause of failure. Hunger is probably the biggest obstacle for most people when they fast for the first time as the body and mind have not yet adjusted to the true nature of hunger. Keep in mind that your body is used to constantly being fed, so the sudden absence of food could well produce signals in your brain that are similar to the fight-or-flight reaction. Your brain tells your body that something must be very wrong because you haven't fed it in several hours. It will likely increase the amount of ghrelin (hunger hormone) that it produces so that you can't miss the message that you "need" to eat now. Work your way through this possibility before you start fasting and get yourself to a point of acceptance. It is important for us to accept and understand that the messages our brain will send us during this initial fast period are essentially false. Try to get to the point where you see past these mixed messages and continually tell yourself that you are simply in transition and that, on the other side of your fast, your brain will start to return to its natural state of true comprehension of the hunger signal. If you have prepared your body with healthy and clean foods in the run-up to your fast, then you consciously know that you have everything you need to get through your water fast.

It is not uncommon to feel lightheaded, dizzy, and sometimes nauseated during your first fast. These are signs that your body is adjusting to a new way of being, and, as you know, a more natural state of being. This is why it is important to ensure that you don't have a lot going on when you plan to fast so that you can rest when you need to deal with these symptoms. Due to the change in food intake, you can also expect your bowel movements to change. There is no need to be alarmed if this happens as it should return to normal fairly quickly. If you are constipated, there is a possibility that you are not drinking enough water, and you should consider increasing your water intake. While we are on the topic of toilet habits, it is possible to drink too much water, and the color of your urine is a good indicator as to whether you are drinking too much or not enough water. Very dark, pungent-smelling urine is an indicator that you are not drinking enough water while completely clear urine means you are drinking too much water. Urine should not have an intense odor, and it should be light in color but tinged yellow.

With regards to weight loss, it is important to have realistic expectations upfront. You are not going to get to your goal weight after one round of fasting. When you fast, your body begins a process of burning through glucose, then fat, and it will become more efficient at doing this, the more you expose it to a fasted state. It is also important to keep in mind that while you may lose pounds on the scale, that does not necessarily equate to body fat. The scale cannot determine what type of weight you are losing, and it is very likely that on your first fast, you will predominantly be losing water weight. Temper your weight loss goals with the acknowledgement that you have started somewhere. Even if you do a 24-hour fast and don't lose a single ounce on the scale, you have initiated processes in your body that are setting you on the right path. Water fasting is not a once-off deal. You need to practice it as a lifestyle in order to get the best benefits from it and that includes weight loss. The way you eat in the run-up to your water fast is also any important part of your weight loss, and if you keep up a healthy diet and clean eating, you will undoubtedly start to shed the extra pounds quickly. Physical activity outside of your fast is also important to encourage weight loss.

Some other side effects that you may experience during fasting include increased body odor as sweating increases to remove toxins from your body, and headaches.

Part of preparing yourself mentally is ensuring that you know why you are doing this. Having a deep visualization of what you want to attain from your fast will help you to keep going when things get rough. For every difficult symptom that you may encounter, there is probably no better adage to keep in mind than "this too shall pass." It really will, and you will likely be surprised at how quickly the negative side effects of fasting do pass. If you are able to keep your goal in mind and continually remind yourself why you decided to fast in the first place, you will be far more likely to succeed. Another great way to prepare yourself mentally is to plan something that you enjoy (not food related obviously) right in the middle of your planned fasting period. A spa day, for instance, is a good example as you will be relaxing and pampering yourself without involving any food.

One of the most important things you will need to do while water fasting is to trust your body. While we like to think that our body and mind are separate, they are not. Our mind does not control our body or vice versa—they work in unison. Your body knows what it needs. This is what we need to learn to trust. Although we may have gotten ourselves to the point as a society where we ignore our body's signals or find ways to mask them so that we don't have to listen, our body continues to communicate its needs. Water fasting is about using your internal intuition to know when to stop and also using your success in fasting to reconnect with your body and begin to trust its judgment again. Perhaps the best explanation of trusting your body is the feeling you get in your gut when you know something is not right. We have all had it, and many of us have ignored it to our peril. Although we ignore the signals that our body gives us, it knows and understands far more than our conscious mind is able to comprehend—we just need to quiet down and listen.

You know yourself better than anyone else, so a big part of successfully preparing yourself for this water fast will be figuring out where you have gone wrong in the past and correcting those mistakes now. Some people cannot be around temptation at all, and if you are one of those people, then in order to succeed, you need to ensure that you keep yourself away from anything or anyone that is going to tempt you to break your fast. Other people may have greater self-discipline in staying away from temptation, but their weakness may be overthinking and creating anxiety for no reason. In your mental preparation phase, ask yourself what you usually do to self-sabotage and what you can do this time to avoid doing so. If you haven't tried any other health regimens before, then you may not have any information about how you react in such situations. If that is the case, then your water fast will be a self-discovery journey as well. Take special note about your emotional reaction to the different parts of the fast, and if you happen to find it difficult to reach your goal the first time round, dig deep to understand why and how you can change that in the future.

Although it is important to push yourself as much as possible and not fall at the first hurdle, you also don't want to do any damage to yourself. As with any other dietary lifestyle or practice, water fasting is not for everyone. If you start to feel very uncomfortable or experience changes in your heart rate or breathing, discontinue your fast immediately and undertake medical advice.

A journal is a really useful tool during this journey as you can use it to record your reasons for wanting to fast, your specific goals, and visualizations. If you are tracking metrics, you can also use it to chart your progress in your fast and how it compares to other water fasts you may do.

5

EVERYTHING YOU NEED TO KNOW ABOUT YOUR WATER FAST

At this point you have prepared your body and your mind for your fast, and you are about to get ready to water fast for the first time. What should you expect to happen in your body and mind while you are fasting? How long should your fast be, and what can you expect to happen at different points during your fast? In this chapter, I will guide you on the completion of a successful water fast from start to finish.

A CHANCE TO RECONNECT

As you begin your water fasting journey, consider this a time to reconnect with your body. You are going to be resetting many of your body's processes and taking yourself out of the unnatural constantly fed state that you are in right now. This is, therefore, the perfect time to build a deeper connection with your body so that, even after your fast ends, you are able to maintain an intuition about what it is that you really need to function at a high level. We spend so much time rushing through life that it is easy to ignore the small changes in our body that actually end up being signs of a deeper issue. When we take time to reconnect with our body and reestablish the connection that stress, anxiety, and modern living has all but severed, we take one of the most important steps toward good health. With the huge increase in the number of pharmaceutical interventions that are now available to us, many of us have reached the stage of answering everything our body tells us with a pill. Headaches are probably one of the most common examples of that. A headache is simply our body telling us that something is happening in our body that we need to pay attention to. It could be that we are dehydrated or stressed, or it could just be a side effect of toxins leaving our body. We simply don't take the time to investigate the cause of these signs our body gives us anymore. Instead, at the first sign of a twinge of pain between the eyes, we pop a tablet. The pain goes away, but it doesn't solve the issue that our body was raising in the first place. Gaining weight and obesity are other signals that our body gives us that we try to ignore in the wrong way. Weight gain is our body's way of telling us that something is wrong, either with the nutrition that we are consuming or at a deeper level within the systems of our body. Instead of undertaking fad diets to just reduce our weight temporarily without addressing the actual issue, water fasting helps us to reset our body so that the issue that originally caused the weight gain is addressed.

It is important to consider your fasting journey as just that—a journey, not a destination. Take the journey slowly and savor every step along the way. This is not a time to rush through, just to get to the other side. If your goal is to get through water fasting just so that you can eat again, then you are already starting with the wrong mindset. There are many things that you can learn about yourself and your body during this time if you allow yourself to.

It is vital to enter into this with the mindset that you are able to start a healing process. We are all born with the ideal and perfect system, but sadly as we get older, we don't always look after our bodies the way we should. Through water fasting, you are looking to reset a lifetime of poor eating habits and overall poor lifestyle, and that is not going to be an easy journey. Just as emotional healing from a trauma means that we have to bring all of the difficult memories to the surface to work through them before we can heal, so does physical healing mean that we are going to have to experience some uncomfortable moments in order to start the healing process. If you want an easy way to achieve this, you will have to wait until such a way is discovered because it doesn't exist yet. Nothing that is worth achieving is easy, and fasting is the same. The benefits that you will receive from fasting are definitely worth the difficulties you may experience during the early days of water fasting. You have to be willing to take it one step at a time. As you fast and feel yourself struggling with one or another part of the fast, try to take the time to interrogate yourself and find out why you are really struggling with that particular element of the fast. This deep self-interrogation could lead to great discoveries about who you are as a person and what you value. This is why it is truly important to practice water fasting when you are in a rested state and you have the ability and time to reflect on your experience and get the most out of it.

As you proceed through your fast, listen to your body and pay attention to how you are feeling. You really know your body better than anyone else, so although you will be experiencing fasting for the first time, if you begin to feel severely ill, rather play it on the safe side and halt your fast. You can always pick it up again at another time, and that is preferable to making yourself really ill.

WHAT TO DRINK AND WHAT NOT TO DRINK

Although it's called water fasting, there are other water-related beverages that you can drink during your fast as long as they contain zero calories. Any intake of calories will immediately stop your fast, so it is vital to ensure that any beverages you take in do not contain any caloric content.

Filtered water is your absolute best option for fasting. You can add a bit of Himalayan or sea salt to the water, which will help you to maintain your electrolyte levels while fasting. A depletion in electrolytes can lead to dizziness, nausea, and headaches, so if you are experiencing any of these symptoms while fasting, you can either add the salt to your water or put a pinch on the back of your tongue. You can also infuse your water with different flavors as long as they are zero calorie. You could use mint, lemon, lime, watermelon, strawberry, or even cucumber to make your water more interesting.

Ensure that you have multivitamins lined up to avoid experiencing any deficiencies and take them every day at the same time. Read the label on the multivitamins you choose to take to ensure that there are no additives which may have a calorie count. Try to avoid caffeinated drinks like black coffee and tea, as although caffeine is thought to stave off hunger, it is also an addictive toxin which will make your fast more difficult. Herbal tea is an excellent alternative as a warm drink; again, depending on the brand you choose, be sure to read the label to ensure the tea has no caloric content. Green tea is possibly one of the most beneficial warm drinks that you can consume while fasting and even when you are not fasting. There are many studies that confirm that green tea is beneficial in weight loss. Green tea contains compounds such as green tea catechins (GTC) and the most powerful of these, concerning weight loss, is epigallocatechin gallate or EGCG. The way in which GTCs aid in weight loss is rather interesting and unexpected. These catechins mimic a state in the body which is similar to our fight-or-flight mode. When we are in this mode, our body releases hormones like noradrenaline which indicate that we need to start burning energy stores at a higher rate in order to give us the strength to either fight or run away. Green tea is particularly beneficial in burning belly fat, which we know is one of the most dangerous forms of fat and also the most difficult to get rid of. A study conducted on participants who had been diagnosed with type 2 diabetes showed that the consumption of green tea helped them to reduce their waist size (reduce belly fat), even though the rest of their body weight was unchanged. This indicates that the GTCs directly target this belly fat above all other types. Another interesting impact of GTCs is that they have been shown to directly reduce levels of ghrelin in the body, thereby making us feel less hungry.

An optimum amount of water to drink, which will vary from person to person, is about 9 to 13 glasses of water. This should be consumed throughout the day to give your body time to absorb it. Drinking too much water at once can make you as ill as drinking too little water. If you feel hunger pangs become quite noticeable, drink a glass of water or two to fill your stomach up and help ease your hunger.

HOW TO DEAL WITH CHALLENGING SIDE EFFECTS

If you prepare yourself beforehand for some of the challenges you may face while fasting, you will be in a far better position to deal with them.

Initially, you may experience some lightheadedness or dizziness while fasting. This could be as a result of your body adjusting to having to use existing energy sources, and if this is the case, it will subside after a nap, which will allow your body to realign its energy usage. Dizziness may also be due to dehydration, so certainly the first thing to do when you begin to feel dizzy is drink a glass or two of water. Make sure that you add a small amount of salt to this water or a pinch on your tongue, as it may also be an electrolyte imbalance which is impacting you.

Another way that you can deal with dizziness is by sitting quietly, closing your eyes, and breathing deeply. Make sure that your in-breath and out-breath are of equal lengths so that you are ridding your lungs of all the carbon dioxide before you take in another breath of oxygen. Continue to do this for a few minutes, focusing not on your lightheadedness but rather on your breathing. Visualizations can also help to make you feel more balanced while you practice deep breathing. With your eyes closed, visualize the oxygen going into your lungs as a stream of white light that is flushing out all of the toxins and then, on the exhale, visualize yourself expelling all of those toxins into the air. This will help you to recenter your thinking on healing and not to focus on the side effects you may be experiencing. If at any time you faint or lose consciousness, stop your fast immediately and consult a doctor.

The reason that we don't recommend you carry out any strenuous acts during your water fast is because, in the initial period at least, beginner fasters are likely to feel quite weak. Your body is undergoing a major transition, and although you may not physically be working out, your cells are having the exercise session of their lives. This weakness will begin to fade and will eventually be replaced by significant energy.

The focus on water in water fasting helps to avoid many of the side effects that people practicing other forms of fasting, such as intermittent fasting (which doesn't have a focus on water consumption), may experience. Headaches, hunger, constipation, and even cravings can all be aided with the consumption of water and electrolytes through salt.

In avoiding your focus on hunger, you can chew on zero-calorie substitutes like fennel seeds or mint leaves. Adding natural hunger busters like cinnamon to your herbal tea is another good option to help stave off hunger pangs. At the root of it, hunger needs to be understood to be conquered during fasting. Hunger, similar to cravings, comes in waves and usually only lasts a few minutes at most. If you can ride out the wave, you can get past the hunger. It simply involves riding out each wave as it comes and not submitting to it. Many people actually have no idea what real hunger feels like. So many of us have bought into the societal ideal of three meals per day that we time our meals by the clock and not by when our body asks for food. Often, we don't even know what it feels like when our body asks for food because it is not our body we are listening to. By approaching your water fast as a journey of discovery, you may find it easier to deal with hunger, or what you think is hunger. Notice how different your so-called hunger alert feels on day one of your fast compared to how it feels on day three of your fast. Also, notice how quickly your body adjusts to not having food because that is its natural state. While your brain may be telling you that you are about to starve to death, your body is wiser than that. Your body understands that it is at no risk at all. It is the mental signals that we need to learn to interpret correctly so that we can tie in the wisdom of our body with the functioning of our minds and the thoughts they create. If you have developed an emotional connection to food, as many of us have without realizing it, you may experience a strange pushback from your brain in the first few days. You may have convinced your brain that food is a reward, a treat, or something you have earned, and when you don't eat, your brain wants to know why you are punishing yourself. You will eventually break this emotional connection to food. Keep reminding yourself that your water fast is your reward. What you are doing is good for you, and it is in no way a punishment. For those who are more analytical, it may be helpful to think of hunger simply as a hormone acting in your body. You know that ghrelin, the hunger hormone, is what is causing your body to feel the way it does. Instead of focusing on the actual feeling of hunger, rather focus your analytical mind, for a few minutes, on picturing how this hormone is working in your body. Acknowledge its presence, thank it for its work, and then drink water to satisfy it. If we are realistic about hunger, we know that the deep gnawing feeling we know as hunger only lasts a few seconds. One or two bites of food would make that feeling disappear completely, and that shows how negligible that feeling is. If one or two bites of food could make the feeling go away, then it is actually quite an easy feeling to ignore and move past.

Some fasting experts suggest having stevia on hand if you were a high sugar consumer prefast. Stevia is a natural sugar replacement which, in most cases, has no caloric content. This is a good way to get a little sweetness into your water without actual sugar or calorie content. Sometimes that is all that is needed to give you a little pick-me-up and urge you forward.

LIFESTYLE CHANGES

In order to get the most out of water fasting, you really need to be willing and able to make some lifestyle changes while you are fasting. I have already indicated the prefast changes that should be made in order to make your fast easier and more successful, and I have outlined the type of activities that you should focus on while you are fasting. The time during which you are fasting really needs to be a self-care period in which you listen to your body and give it what it needs in terms of rest and hydration.

It is important to avoid stress as much as possible during fasting, and if you plan to exercise, keep it to light exercises like yoga and stretching. If you start to feel really faint and drained about halfway through your fast, you can try drinking a bit of bone broth, which will provide you with salts and minerals to replenish your electrolytes. For vegetarians or vegans, instant miso soup from your local health shop will be a perfect replacement. If this is insufficient, try eating a small piece of raw fruit if absolutely necessary. Rather than push yourself to the point of really not enjoying a water fast the first time round, break early if you need to and then you can work your way up on your next fast. There has to be a first time for everything, and really, it's about gaining the experience of your first water fast so that you can build on that and gain the confidence to grow in your fasting journey.

When you start including water fasting as a regular event in your life, it is a good idea to schedule it sometime in advance so that you can allocate your preparation time and really set yourself up for success. While water fasting is a very individual exercise, encouragement and bonding with others can be beneficial, especially when you are new to water fasting. There are quite a few online forums, especially on social media, in which water fasting is a hot topic. While you may find great support on such forums, also ensure that you research and verify any information that is provided by members of the public.

Curiosity can be a very rewarding trait, and your water fasting journey is a great time to develop curiosity about your body and its response to certain conditions. Rather than relying on the studies of others, use your water fasting journey to create some of your own research and, in so doing, learn more about how your body works. You can track various metrics to measure your progress and response along the way. By doing this, you can also have peace of mind about what is happening in your body. Some of the metrics you can consider tracking include:

- ketones
- pH balance
- cholesterol
- liver function
- iron levels
- vitamin D levels
- body measurements
- body fat percentage
- weight
- muscle mass percentage
- body water percentage

You don't need to go to the doctor every time you want to test one of these metrics. You can purchase home testing kits for all of the above-mentioned metrics online to track your progress in the comfort of your own home. To get good data, start tracking these metrics before you even begin your preparation phase. You can record these on a computer or in a notebook. If you are conducting an initial 24-hour fast, test yourself before you start your preparation, then once in the middle of your fast, once after your postfast period, and wait a few days after you resume your normal eating routine and test yourself again. In this way, you don't need to guess as to the difference that water fasting is having on your body or rely on how you feel. You can have facts in number form right in front of you. While each individual will differ, the following are the average acceptable ranges for the metrics you may test:

- Ketones: you will be in ketosis if your reading is 1.5 to 3.0 mmol/l
- pH balance: normal pH level of the human body is 7.40
- Cholesterol: LDL cholesterol levels should be less than 100mg/dL
- Liver function: AST liver function is normal at 10-40 units per liter, and ALT liver function is normal at 7-56 per liter
- Iron levels: 35.5-44.9%
- Vitamin D levels: 20-50 ng/mL
- Body measurements: per individual
- Body fat percentage: 21-33% in women and 8-19% in men
- Weight: per individual
- Muscle mass percentage: this is highly dependent on age and gender, but in general, a good range is between 30.4 and 35.1% for women and between 39.4 and 44% for men
- Body water percentage: 45-65%

By measuring these metrics, you can also see what works for you as an individual and what doesn't. If you are unsure about what might break your fast and you are getting conflicting information in your research, test it out by measuring your ketones before and after.

By really drilling down into these measurable metrics, you will be able to gain a factual basis for your standpoint on water fasting. If the tests and readings all seem a bit overwhelming, choose the ones that will align best with your goals. If you are trying to lose weight, you will want to know if you are going into fat burning so make testing your ketones a priority.

6

THE POSTFAST PERIOD

Just as the way in which you start your fast and the things you do while you are fasting are important, the way you end your fast is vital. By ending your fast in the wrong way, you can actually undo a lot of the good you have done, and in the worst-case scenario, you can make yourself ill. Breaking your water fast is almost a reverse of the actions you took when you started your fast, and it encourages a seamless transition back into your normal routine. The longer you have fasted for, the more important a gradual breaking of the fast becomes.

In one of the most common religious fasts, the Muslim fast of Ramadan, it has been noted that followers commonly break their fast with a small meal. They will then attend a prayer service for the evening and only after they return will they enjoy a full meal. This type of fasting is very different from water fasting and is more in line with intermittent fasting, but the slow breaking of the fast is applicable even here and outlines its importance. In research that has been undertaken around followers of the Ramadan fast, those who do not break their fast in such a way, and instead launch into a huge meal to break their fast, report feeling ill, gaining weight, and experiencing severe indigestion. Due to the fact that water fasting is so much more intense than this type of religious fasting and, in most cases, much longer, the breaking of the fast becomes all the more important.

Another common mistake is thinking that as soon as your water fast ends, you can immediately start with strenuous activity and resume your normal routine immediately. Just as your body needs time to ease into water fasting, it also needs time to ease out.

RESTARTING YOUR DIGESTIVE SYSTEM

Depending on how long you have water fasted for on this occasion, you must be consciously aware of the fact that you have essentially halted your digestive process for the entire time that you have been fasting. The production of gastric juices has mostly stopped, and your digestive system is going to be sluggish to begin with. Consider a vehicle that has been standing for a long time. You wouldn't jump in, rev the engine ferociously, and immediately race off down the road, would you? Instead, you would start the engine and let it run for a while, allowing it to heat up before racing away with it. By the same token, your digestive system must be restarted slowly. If you immediately flood your digestive system with a huge amount of foods that are difficult to digest, it is almost always going to struggle to digest that food properly.

When you break a fast, you are rebuilding your digestive system, which includes your gut and stomach lining. Breaking a fast too quickly will result in toxins being created in your body, and you will have wasted the time you spent fasting. A baby does not come out of the womb munching down on a cheeseburger and fries. We start infants off with a liquid diet and slowly work them up to solids. A similar process applies to coming out of a fast.

Ideally, break your fast with a glass of fruit juice, preferably one that you have prepared at home so that you avoid the high amounts of sugar that are often in store-bought juices. Orange and lime juice are good options, and you can add a spoonful of honey to it if necessary. A light vegetable soup or a glass of coconut water is also a good way to break your fast, with the latter containing a huge amount of beneficial electrolytes. Wait about half an hour for this initial consumption to digest and see how you feel. If you feel a little ill, wait a bit longer to move on to the next step. If you feel fine, you can move onto a fruit smoothie. Again, give your body time to digest this smoothie. Preferably, don't spend this time focused on food and thinking about what you are going to eat next. Instead, continue with a low-stress activity and try to keep your mind off food. In a few hours, if you are feeling well and your stomach is not bloated or uncomfortable, you can eat a small amount of fermented food such as sauerkraut or a source of healthy fat like avocado. Although kefir is a very popular fermented food, it is not good for breaking a water fast as it is dairy based in origin and, therefore, more difficult to digest.

Keep in mind that you need to apply as much discipline in breaking your fast as you did in your preparation and during your water fast. The general rule is that your postfast recovery should be the same number of days over which your fast lasted. If you fasted for 24 hours, then you should not eat a full meal until 24 hours after ending your fast. This also depends on the individual. If you are an otherwise healthy individual with a normally strong digestive system, you could break your fast a bit quicker, but if you suffer from health conditions and usually have a sluggish digestive system, you may want to take it even slower. As with all other stages of a water fast, listen to your body and take it slow.

It is important not to let your guard down at the point of breaking your fast. You have done such good work so far and worked hard to give your body this natural reset, so it would be a pity to see all of that hard work go to waste by allowing yourself to slip back into your normal routine immediately. Guard your mental and emotional state at this time, as well, as your brain will likely be telling you to go back to your usual food routine. It is important to consider how good your normal routine was to begin with. One of the most exciting parts about fasting is that you have essentially wiped your nutritional slate clean. If you have ever wanted to eat a better diet, now is the time to do so. If you have been wanting to switch over to a plant-based diet, for instance, your body and mind are now in the prime state to make that change. Consider this as you ease back into eating as your "normal" routine is very likely not the best to revert back to. In terms of exercise, if your usual routine involves strenuous exercise, don't get back into this for at least a week after you have resumed normal eating. Instead practice yoga, stretch, and take short walks. Just as you build up your eating, you should also build up the exercise and activity you do, slowly and progressively to avoid overexerting yourself.

When we return to eating after a fast, there is a significant possibility of reactive weight gain if we immediately return to a diet of processed and unhealthy foods. It would be unfortunate to work hard during a fast to cleanse your body and possibly lose weight only to pick up additional weight after a water fast simply because you have gone back to an unhealthy diet.

SAMPLE FAST-BREAKING DAY

How you break your water fast is very important and, as such, it is important to remove any confusion about exactly what you should eat and when during your postfast period. As an example of how a fast should be broken, I will lay out an eating guide which you can use in order to break your fast. This guide will work on the presumption that you have undertaken a 72-hour (3-day) fast, but if you have only fasted for 24 hours, you can still apply the same idea, just over a shorter period. Feel free to switch up the ingredients to items that you are able to get or that are affordable for you.

Day One

This is the first day of eating after your fast. Your digestive system is very sensitive on this day, and it is important to take it slow and ensure you don't overdo it. On this day, you will not take in any solid food. Start with a glass of fruit juice, a small cup of vegetable soup, bone broth, or coconut water. Do not take in any dairy product on this day as they are very difficult to digest and will disturb your digestive system. Essentially, what you want to eat today is just one step up from water—a liquid that contains some calories but preferably more nutrients.

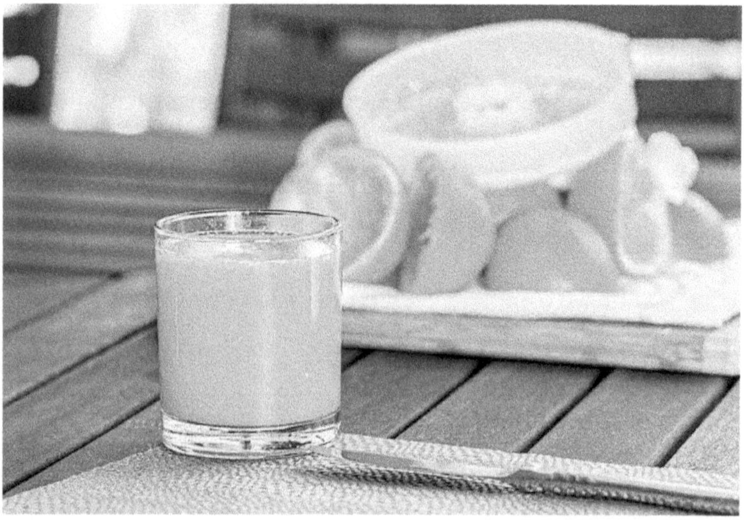

Don't jump into any strenuous activities right away either. Give your body time to adjust to the fact that you are feeding it again. Your digestive system is slowly starting up. Consume your food slowly at all times. With today's liquid diet, sip slowly and give the body time to move the liquid down to your stomach before taking another sip. Gulping down your first liquid meal is going to make you feel rather ill, and you will enjoy it far more if you consume it slowly.

Day Two

Today you can move on to light and easily digested solids. Good options for today would include papaya, avocado, watermelon, cantaloupe, and ripe banana. Have some of these fruits in the morning and pay attention to how your digestive system reacts. This will be a good indication of whether you are moving too fast. If you feel ill or uncomfortable or begin to vomit when you first take in solid foods, revert back to liquid for another day as your digestive system needs more time to adjust. If you ingest these fruits in the morning or early afternoon and feel well, you can prepare a plate of boiled vegetables as an early dinner. Potato is an easily digestible starch vegetable for this meal but eat only a small portion. Cruciferous vegetables like broccoli, cauliflower, and brussels sprouts are difficult to digest, so they should be avoided. Vegetables that are easy to digest include yellow squash, pumpkin, spinach, beets, green beans, and carrots. Don't eat too late in the day when you are breaking your fast as our metabolism naturally slows down when we sleep, and you want to ensure that you have digested your food properly before you go to sleep.

Remember to chew your food really well so that you help your digestive system to get going again. In general, most people do not chew their food sufficiently and also eat far too quickly. This results in us consuming more food than we need because we are missing the full signal in our brains. It also results in indigestion, which is almost like traffic congestion for your digestive system. If you let everything in at once, your body doesn't have time to move it down to your stomach, and you will end up feeling like half your meal is stuck in your esophagus.

Day Three

Today you can have your first solid meal. It is preferable to only eat one such meal in the day, and the best time is around midday to allow for full digestion. Keep your portions small and avoid any processed foods. Don't include any spice in your food and try to stick to foods like rice, wheat, or oats. An excellent option would be a bowl of cooked oats with ripe banana. Other good options include eggs, avocado, nuts, and spinach. Stick to soft foods for a while and definitely avoid meat for as long as you can after you have completed your fast.

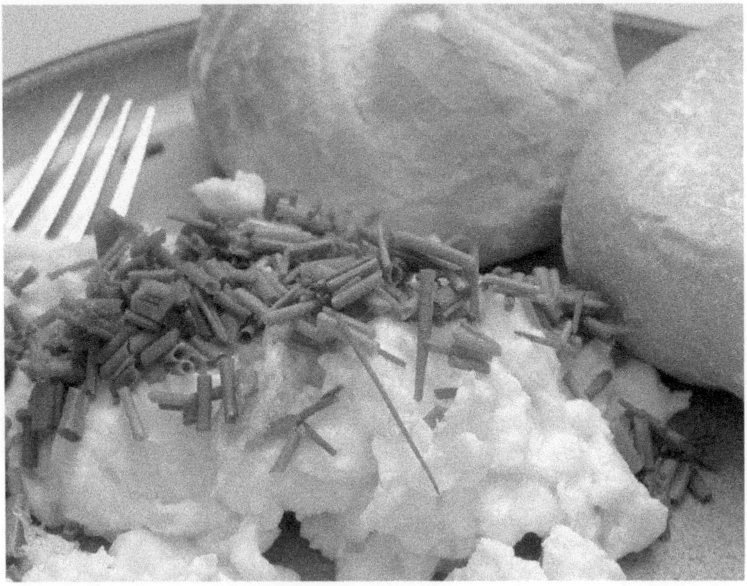

For the rest of the day, continue with fruit juices, smoothies, and boiled vegetables. Pay close attention to how you are feeling after you eat this meal both physically and emotionally. If you feel that you have moved too quickly, revert back to day one or two and start again. You literally cannot move too slowly in breaking your fast. While raw foods might sound healthier, they are also more difficult to digest, and it's not recommended within your immediate postfast period. Another ideal first meal may be a scrambled egg with soft cooked vegetables and a few cubes of avocado.

Day Four Onward

Slowly increase your number of meals and portions until you are eating a well-rounded, balanced diet again. Again, try to use this period of readjustment to make changes to your diet that you have always wanted to. This period is also very important in understanding the hidden obsessions with foods that may exist in our psyche. By taking this breaking of fast slowly, you can pay attention, not just to your physical body but also to what is happening in your mind as you reintroduce food into your routine. Remember to chew properly and don't eat too quickly. By doing this, you will also find that you feel fuller quicker as you give your body time to recognize that it is receiving food and register fullness.

Once you have completed your fast, consider what foods you really missed. If you didn't particularly miss eating meat, for instance, this might be the ideal time to cut it out entirely. While lean meat is a good source of protein in moderation, when eaten too often it can cause a myriad of health issues. In increasing the amount of fruit and vegetables that you eat, keep in mind that it doesn't have to be fresh to be healthy. In the past frozen fruit and vegetables held only a small portion of the nutrients that the fresh option did. Freezing technology in the food industry has grown significantly, though, and today, there are just as many nutrients in the frozen option. Fruit can also be kept frozen for smoothies, which are not just easy on the digestive system but a great way to include a wide variety of fruits and vegetables in your diet.

When restructuring your postfast diet, stay away from low-fat products. This may sound counterintuitive, but the low-fat fad that once swept the food market has started to make way for full-fat options again as people have realized the deception behind the low-fat label. When manufacturers make products "low-fat," they have to include something else in the product to make up for the missing fat, and what they usually include is carbohydrates. If you carefully compare the label of a low-fat yogurt, for example, compared to a full-fat or medium-fat product, you will see that the carbohydrate level on the low-fat option is far higher. These are also not good carbohydrates that are easily digested by your body; they are refined carbohydrates.

Another small adjustment that you can make to your diet which will have a big impact is to use fresh herbs in your cooking. Buy bunches of fresh herbs and store them in your fridge with the stems in a glass of water. In this way, you can keep them fresh for up to two weeks and just snip off what you would like as you go. Fresh herbs are a fantastic source of natural medicinal properties. At the same time, keep a head of ginger and a bulb of turmeric root in your freezer for the same reason. These can be grated from frozen into food. The following are some examples of healthy herbs and spices that you should use more often in cooking:

- Turmeric: excellent in curries and a powerful anti-inflammatory when paired with a fat like coconut oil and black pepper.
- Cinnamon: helps to reduce blood sugar levels, stave off hunger, and has a powerful antidiabetic effect.

- Sage: has been used to great effect in research trials with Alzheimer's Disease patients and helps to improve brain function and memory.
- Peppermint: helps to relieve pain from irritable bowel syndrome and aids in treating nausea.
- Basil: excellent in Italian dishes and also helps fight infections and boost immunity.
- Cayenne pepper: helps to reduce appetite and has cancer-fighting properties.
- Ginger: also fabulous in curries and can treat nausea and has anti-inflammatory properties.
- Fenugreek: has beneficial effects in leveling out blood sugar.
- Rosemary: prevents nasal congestion and allergies
- Garlic: contains allicin which combats illness and improves heart health. (Tip: when cooking with fresh garlic, don't cut and cook immediately. Peel the clove and then crush and allow to sit for a few minutes before cooking. This gives the allicin time to build up to its highest levels.)

It is important to understand the difference in various fats as well, as the word has become synonymous with something bad in the last few decades, and that is really not the case. We need fats in our diet, but we need the right fats. There are two types of fats in general: saturated and unsaturated fats. Saturated fats are bad for us. They are found in processed meats and junk food. Unsaturated fats are good for us and we need them. An example of this is omega-3 that is found in wild-caught salmon. It is just as unhealthy to cut out all of the good fats in our diet as it is to include too many bad fats. From a cooking oil perspective, plant-based oils are generally unsaturated except for the tropical oils like coconut and palm oil.

One of the greatest things about water fasting is that it doesn't require a range of expensive and exotic foods in order to accomplish the goal. Many of the fad diets we see call for some of the wildest ingredients and wilder still, is what those ingredients cost. Water fasting is accessible to everyone because it doesn't cost anything, and you will actually end up saving money because you won't be eating during your fast. Feel free to structure your postfast eating to food available in your region and that suits your budget. We spend a lot of time thinking about, preparing, and eating food, and you will likely be pleasantly surprised by how much time and money you save when you fast.

REFEEDING SYNDROME

A slow reintroduction of food into the system after water fasting is so vital as there is a specific syndrome that can develop if a person who has experienced an extended period without food suddenly gorges on huge amounts of solid food. While this syndrome is far more common in people who have suffered from eating disorders or who have not voluntarily stopped eating, it is important to understand what the syndrome entails. The slow progression into and out of a water fast is the difference between a healthy reset of your digestive system and other body processes and a possibly damaging experience.

Refeeding syndrome is seen when food is too quickly reintroduced to people who have experienced an absence of nutrition for a protracted period. It is characterized by the sudden production of glycogen, protein, and fat, which leads to low concentrations of minerals such as phosphorus, magnesium, and potassium in the blood. The pulmonary and cardiac systems can be affected, and the person may even experience neurological symptoms. When insulin production is forced to resume in the body at an accelerated rate, the increase of the synthesis of macronutrients uses up the minimal mineral stores far too quickly, and when these stores are so quickly depleted, it can have devastating effects on the body.

While refeeding syndrome is extremely rare in those coming out of water fasting, it is important to understand the impact that it can have on the body so that exceptional emphasis is placed on the postfast period.

7

OTHER COMMON QUESTIONS ABOUT WATER FASTING

In this chapter, I will answer some of the questions that you still may have around water fasting that have not yet been addressed. As water fasting has become more popular, several myths have sprung up around the practice, and it is important to address those. By fully educating yourself around water fasting and entering into the practice with no doubts or questions, you can experience a safe and beneficial fast.

How Long Can I Fast For?

The human body can go for about a month without food. Such a period for fasting is neither necessary nor healthy, though, as you can glean the same benefits from shorter periods. The "slow and steady" approach cannot be emphasized enough. There is no benefit for a first-time faster to enter into a 7-day fast. Not only will you likely fail, but it will be a very difficult and uncomfortable experience. If you have never fasted before, start with 24 hours or less. Once you have achieved a full 24-hour water fast and you feel comfortable and well, you can consider working your way up. Eventually you could build yourself up to 7 to 14 days of water fasting if your lifestyle allows for this. Keep in mind that the period that you choose to actually fast in must be multiplied by three in order to calculate how much time you actually need for the prefast and postfast activities. For an active, relatively healthy person, a 72-hour fast once per month is ideal. Studies have also shown that age can impact the length for which you can safely fast. The general rule of thumb is that the higher your nutritional needs at a particular stage of life, the shorter your fast should be. It is for this reason that children under the age of 18 should not fast at all as they need high levels of nutrition to grow. Young adults are often still in bone and brain development and can handle shorter fasts. The optimum age group to start longer fasting is around 40. At this age, your nutritional requirements are lower, and you are able to handle going without food for longer periods. As we age, we can fast for even longer periods. If you suffer from health conditions or you are overweight, you can consider going for a longer fast on several occasions throughout the year, but you should always consult a doctor first.

Why Do I Experience Unpleasant Side Effects While Fasting?

The irony of toxins is that they feel great going in and horrendous coming out. Processed and junk food tastes delicious, smoking is a pleasurable addiction for some, and alcohol consumption seems fun and casual while you are doing it. The toxins that these things create in our body, though, are so bad for us that when we undergo a process like water fasting to rid our bodies of them, we tend to feel ill while it's happening. The process of healing and detoxification can, unfortunately, be uncomfortable, but it is not only very necessary but highly beneficial in the long run. Symptoms of detoxification during a water fast can include dizziness, nausea, diarrhea, and skin breakouts or a change in skin composition. While these side effects are not pleasant, they should never make you feel violently ill or lose consciousness. Detoxification from severe toxins like hard drugs is done under medical supervision only because it is a very dangerous process. If you feel like your body is reacting very severely to a normal detoxification process while water fasting, you should stop immediately and see a doctor.

Will I Lose Muscle Mass When I Fast?

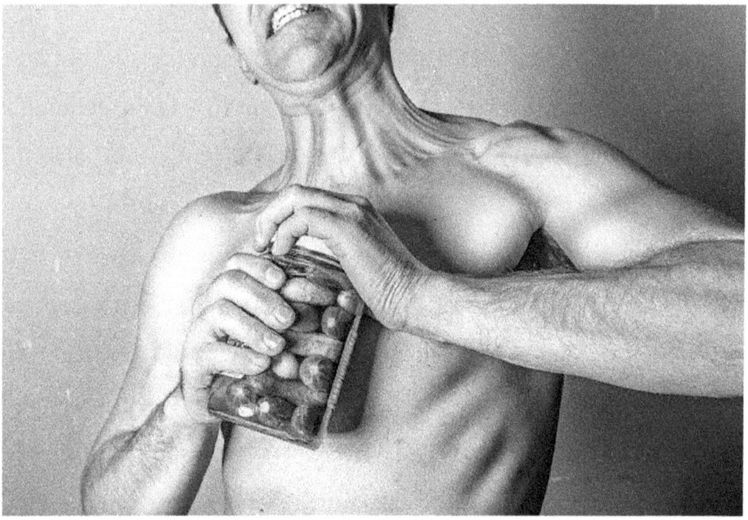

The short answer to this question is when done correctly water fasting should never cause the loss of muscle mass. Losing muscle mass is certainly not an aim of water fasting, and it is not beneficial to our body. When we water fast, we aim to first work through our glucose stores and then move onto our fat deposits. Depending on the length of your fast, most of your weight loss will come from water weight, and while you will feel leaner, there will be no reduction in your muscle mass. Fasting actually promotes the production of human growth hormone which plays a significant role in the production of muscle tissue. The higher levels of human growth hormone in your blood will also work to protect your muscles from wastage.

Will I Regain the Weight I Lost After My Fast Ends?

The possibility of regaining weight depends on the type of weight you have lost while water fasting. If you have done a 24-hour fast, then you have likely lost water weight, and this will be regained when you resume your normal food consumption. Research shows that you may lose up to two pounds per day during a 24-hour to 72-hour fast, but much of the initial weight will be water weight. If you have moved past your glucose stores and started burning fat, however, that weight loss can be maintained with the correct postfast activities. If you break your fast correctly and continue to eat a healthy, balanced diet when your fasting is complete, you have a far greater chance of maintaining your weight loss. Remember that in your few initial fasts, weight loss should not be the main goal. Instead, you should be focused on getting your body used to water fasting so that you can undertake longer fasts in which you will lose more weight. You are also resetting your digestive system and food consumption habits during fasting, so while you may not lose a huge amount of weight during the actual fast, the changes in your body and lifestyle thereafter could aid in additional weight loss.

How Can I Deal With Headaches While Fasting?

Headaches experienced during water fasting can be a result of a wide variety of causes. The most common reason you develop headaches while fasting is due to dehydration, and this is a sign that you have not increased your water consumption enough to make up for the fluid that you would usually get from food. In order to remove toxins, your body needs water, and if there is insufficient water available to get rid of the level of toxins that need to be expelled, they will start to build up in your system. This build will cause, among other symptoms, headaches. If you start to feel a headache building, immediately drink one or two glasses of water. If this is indeed the cause of your headache, the pain will start to ease within half an hour. If you do not receive relief from drinking water, you can also try putting a pinch of salt on the back of your tongue. This will help to replenish your electrolytes. Peppermint oil is known to provide relief for headaches, and this is certainly something you should try. Peppermint oil can be used by placing a few drops in your bath. You can also pour hot water into a bowl, add a few drops of peppermint oil to the water, cover your head and the bowl with a towel, and inhale and exhale deeply into the steam. Do this for about two minutes. You could also make peppermint tea by steeping peppermint leaves in hot water for a few minutes. Do not ingest peppermint essential oil unless it is food grade and, even then, only if it is zero calorie. When fasting, medication for headaches should always be a last resort. It is not good to take medication on an empty stomach, and if you develop a headache or migraine to such an extent that you cannot relieve it with any of the aforementioned tips or a nap, you may want to consider ending your fast instead and trying again at a later stage.

What Can I Do About Heartburn While Fasting?

In the initial stages of your fast, you may experience heartburn as your stomach hasn't entirely stopped producing gastric acids yet, but it also doesn't have any food to work on. This may result in a burning sensation in your chest or near your diaphragm. For some people this may be the first time they have experienced heartburn, and it could be a rather alarming sensation. Warm water works well to reduce heartburn. To help during the day, start the morning off with a glass of warm water, which should be slowly sipped and not gulped all at once. It may also help to take a nap while keeping your head elevated and your upper body propped up.

If you suffer from severe heartburn or gastroesophageal reflux disorder, you may want to consider intermittent rather than water fasting as when the stomach is empty and continues to make stomach acid for long periods, this can lead to a worsening of the condition.

What Could Happen to My Bowel Movements While I Am Fasting?

The impact of water fasting on bowel movements is quite an individual experience. You may experience constipation, you may experience no need to have a bowel movement at all, or you may experience diarrhea. All of these instances are normal and depend on how you have prepared your body for the fast as well as how many toxins you need to remove from your body. Your bowel movement is one of the ways that your body uses to remove waste products and toxins from your food that are left over after food has been digested. It stands to reason that if you are not taking in any food, then there is nothing to come out, so if you don't feel the need to have a bowel movement at all, you needn't be concerned. If you ordinarily are not very regular or you haven't prepared very well in the run-up to your fast, then you may find that you become constipated as you may still have some fecal matter left in your bowel when you start fasting, and due to the changes in your digestive system, your body struggles to get that out. In this case, try to increase your water intake slightly as this can help you to move your bowels. If constipation becomes painful or very uncomfortable, you can try using a mild laxative suppository after consulting a doctor. In some cases, your body will use your bowel to cleanse itself of all the toxins it is cleaning out, and you may experience diarrhea. The stool in this case may be strange in color or odor, but you should not be alarmed unless you see any blood in your stool. If you do develop diarrhea, be sure to increase your water intake as you will be losing a lot of water with your stool which will need to be replenished to avoid developing dehydration.

How Often Can I Do a Water Fast?

Beginners can fast for 24 hours once per week but keep in mind that this involves an extra two days—one before and one after—for prefast and postfast activities. If you are able to allocate three days per week to the type of environment that it takes to water fast properly, then you can do that. You could elect to fast every second weekend as you will likely not be working or attending college at that time, and you can undertake a 24-hour fast properly. Once you feel that you are getting used to fasting and 24 hours is becoming relatively easy to accomplish, you can not only start to increase the period that you fast but also increase the gap in between fasts. So, as your next level up, for instance, you could do a three-day fast once per month or once every two months. As water fasting becomes part of your lifestyle, you will start to feel when your body needs to fast again, and you can then find an appropriate period of time in your schedule to do so. If you are experiencing a great deal of stress but also feel like your body needs a water fast, rather try an intermittent fast or simply eat clean and whole foods instead of conducting a proper water fast. When the period of stress has passed, then you can water fast again. There is no set schedule for the number of times you should fast per week, month, or year as every individual is different. In all cases, start small and work your way up. You will get great benefit from any amount of fasting, and studies show that just one 24-hour period of fasting per month can reduce your risk of heart attack by up to 40% (Water Fasting, 2020).

Is Water Fasting Safe for Women?

Much has been said about the delicate balance of various hormones in a woman's body and the possibility that fasting of any nature could put these out of balance. There is no scientific evidence to prove that water fasting has any negative impact on the sex hormones in a woman's body. In fact, water fasting is ideal for menopausal and postmenopausal women as it helps to balance out the levels of estrogen in their body and increase the levels of hormones which naturally start to decrease with age, including human growth hormone and brain-derived neurotrophic factor. Women who are trying to conceive, already pregnant, or breastfeeding should not practice water fasting until they have moved through this time. It is also probably not advisable for women to water fast at the same time as their menstrual period. This has nothing to do with hormone levels, though, and it is more a matter of convenience and comfort. Women can already feel rather unwell during their menstrual period so to add the pressure of fasting onto that would not be a good idea. Studies have shown that women actually tend to do slightly better on water fasts than men because their energy requirements are smaller.

Why Do I Feel Bloated When I Start Eating Again?

If you experience bloating when you start eating again after a fast, then you have likely started with solids too quickly. As each digestive system is different, even if you only did a 24-hour fast and started eating solids within the recommended 24-hour period after your fast, it may simply be too soon for your body. Go back to juices and smoothies and slowly work your way back up to solid food.

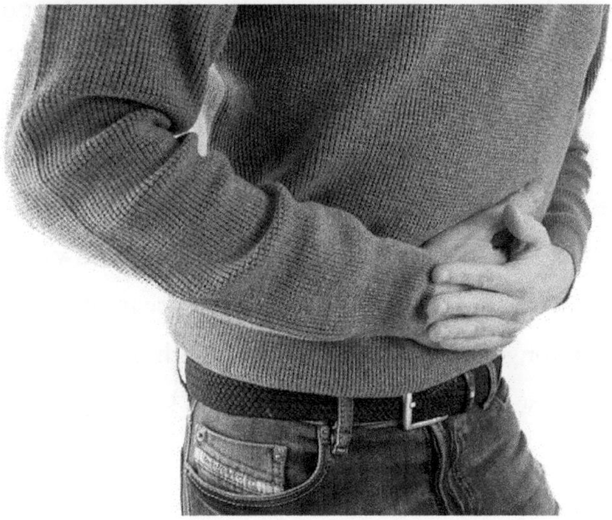

The types of food you eat, in general, can also add to bloating, but that is not always a bad thing. Some foods are not broken down by gastric acid; instead, they sit in your gut and are fermented by your gut bacteria. This fermentation process releases gases which can cause bloating and flatulence, but this process is actually very good for your gut. By providing your gut bacteria with foods that contain resistant starches such as beans and cruciferous vegetables, you are giving your bacteria a bit of exercise which helps to strengthen them. Your body also absorbs nutrients better through this fermentation process.

What Can I Do About Bad Breath While Fasting?

You may experience a reaction to fasting which is commonly referred to as "detox tongue." Basically, it is a build-up of white substance on the tongue which is a part of the detoxification process. Not everyone gets this side effect, but for those who do, it can be quite annoying. Other than brushing your teeth frequently and using a tongue scraper, you can also chew on mint leaves or gargle with a diluted solution of food-grade hydrogen peroxide. Be careful with store-bought mouthwash as it can contain hidden calories. Besides the accumulation of toxins on the tongue, a bad taste in your mouth or bad breath can also be caused by the larger quantity of ketones in your system. People who practice a Keto diet will be familiar with the fruity smell of the breath which is called Keto breath. This happens when we fast, too, as our ketone level increases. The best ways around this, without breaking our fast, is to brush your teeth regularly and increase your intake of water.

My Family is Concerned—How Can I Convince Them?

When people don't understand something, they tend to fear it. So, your best bet is to share the facts with them. If they are open minded, the research and data that are presented in this book and in other resources should allay their fears. Sometimes people just don't want to be convinced, though, and that's okay. If you are over the age of 18 (which you should be to water fast anyway), you don't need anyone's permission to try something new for your health. Family members or friends who are skeptical beforehand will likely be less so when they see the results at the end of your water fast. Family members who live with you are probably concerned about what your practice of fasting will mean for them. In such a case, be clear that all you need from them is to not purposefully make it more difficult for you. Explain that you do not expect them to join in water fasting and that they are more than welcome to continue with life as normal. You may want to point out the benefits that your water fasting will bring for them too. You will have more energy, you will be healthier, and you will live longer. These are all things that any loving family member or friend should value.

Can I Brush My Teeth While Fasting?

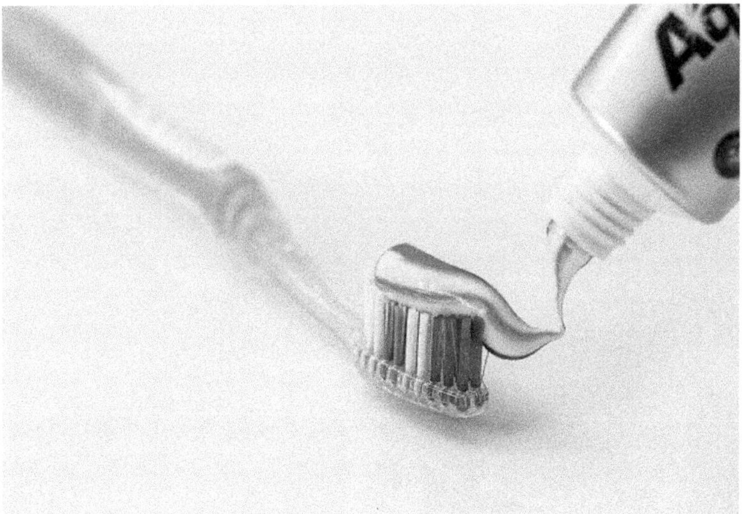

The question of whether brushing your teeth and the possible intake of a small amount of toothpaste would break the fast is often raised. Even though you are not eating, it is still a good idea to continue with your oral hygiene as you may be collecting toxins on your tongue while you sleep resulting in an unpleasant taste in your mouth as well as a bit of bad breath. Depending on the brand of your toothpaste and what it contains, there is a very good chance that it will not break your fast. Read the ingredients to be sure, but the small amount of toothpaste that you may ingest while brushing will likely have almost no effect on insulin levels.

CONCLUSION

For millions of years, humans ate when they had access to food. Sometimes that would be once a week, and sometimes that would be once a month. It's only been in the last few centuries, since the agricultural revolution, that we really started to build the idea of a constantly fed society. Of course, there have been significant benefits to this change. We no longer die of hunger, we don't suffer from undernutrition as much as we used to, and many nutrition-based diseases, like scurvy, have been almost completely eliminated. We are also very different in body structure now, and our energy needs are significantly different. These differences in lifestyle, though, do not account for the enormous difference in the way we eat. There has been a significant downside to this eat-on-demand culture, and now, the world's greatest nutrition-based problems are overnutrition and obesity.

As a result of this increase in obesity and the chronic illnesses which have come with it, we have seen a corresponding marked increase in the number of "quick-fix" solution fad diets. The problem with these fad diets is that they have very little basis in science, and they also do not have much social proof in terms of members of the public who have followed the diet and can say that 20 years later for instance, they've had no negative effects from it. The other problem with these diets is that all they do is help you lose weight—there are no other health benefits. Fasting, and in particular, water fasting, is the only overall weight loss and health regimen that has thousands of years of social proof. It is also the only one with significant clinical studies having been conducted which provide data to support its claimed benefits.

Despite all of these phenomenal benefits and historical significance, water fasting is not for everyone. In this book, I have clearly expressed the situations and circumstances under which water fasting is not the ideal practice. Should you have any doubts about whether water fasting would be good for you, please consult your doctor before making the decision.

I wrote this book because water fasting made an enormous difference in my life, and I wanted to share not just my experience but also the knowledge that I have gained through my studies and my patients' fasting experiences. Knowledge and research is absolutely key if you are considering water fasting because if you don't follow the correct procedures, you can not only make yourself rather ill but you may also waste your time as you could undo any benefits you gained during your fasting period. This book has covered the water fasting journey from beginning to end, providing you with the necessities for prefast preparation, the experience you can expect from the actual fasting period, as well as how to safely end your fast.

As transparency is vital in matters of health, I have also provided you with details of the clinical studies in which many of the benefits of water fasting have been proven. The links to these studies are contained in the references section, and I encourage you to view those studies yourself and also to do further research, if required, until you feel satisfied that you have done due diligence in researching the practice of water fasting.

Water fasting is not a quick-fix solution. It is a lifestyle, and once you immerse yourself in it, it becomes a phenomenal tool for improving your health both physically and mentally. I think that one of the reasons that I connected so deeply with water fasting—and I have no doubt that you will too—is that it truly is a holistic regimen. When I undertake a water fast, I don't just come out the other side a few pounds lighter. I come out rejuvenated in every way. I am a really curious person, and because I struggled so much with my health in my youth, I probably find it more interesting than many others do, to understand exactly how my body works.

In order to really gain the full array of benefits from water fasting, it is important to set time aside for the practice. It's really not something that you want to squeeze in between work and socializing, for instance. The true healing from water fasting happens when you allow yourself to simply be and provide yourself with space to recover from the difficulties of life and expel the toxins from your body that have built up over the years.

If I think about how much money the anti-ageing industry is worth—the creams, the potions, the "magic" elixirs—it is quite amazing to think that the true secret to real cellular-level anti-ageing has always been inside us, and it's free! I am excited to see what the medical community does with the revelations that have recently been made around autophagy. Its applications in disease prevention and treatment are almost endless. The most wonderful thing about the discovery of this process and its applications in our body is that we don't have to wait for permission to use it. The process has always belonged to us, and now we know how to trigger it so that no matter what our age, through water fasting we can benefit from the renewal properties of autophagy. The knowledge that we gain in learning about autophagy and water fasting and its benefits is really empowering. Most of us dread old age as we have been made to believe that we have no choice but to tumble down into a pit of illness and health difficulties. Along with that, we have been made to believe that we have no control over the fact that we will lose our cognitive abilities as we age. For some, that thought is more frightening than any other. With the knowledge we have gained in the arena of ageing in the last few years, though, we now realize that this inevitable doom of old age is simply not accurate. We can control how we age to a great extent, and we don't have to resign ourselves to suffering as we get older. By using water fasting to trigger autophagy in our body, we can make every effort to prevent chronic disease, obesity, and premature death. We just have to be willing to put in a bit of work and commitment.

As we near the end of the book, I would like to request that if the experience and knowledge that I have shared with you in *Water Fasting: How to Lose Weight Fast, Increase Mental Clarity, Heal Your Body, & Activate Autophagy With Water Fasting*, has been beneficial to you, that you pass this knowledge on too. The best way to do this is by giving the book a positive review on Amazon so that others can find the book and benefit from it too. There is truly no greater feeling than knowing that you have helped another human being to avoid the difficulties that you may have experienced. It's why I wrote this book, and it's why I am asking you to share this book. In your reviews, I would also love to hear about your water fasting experience so that we can learn and grow from the journeys of others.

Most importantly, as you start your water fasting journey, I hope that your experience will be as beneficial as mine was. We all have regrets, on occasion, about things we wish we could have done differently, especially from a health perspective. Water fasting is your chance to correct those missteps. It's a reset on our digestive system, and to a large extent, on our lifestyle. This practice is not just about losing weight. It is about using the processes that already exist in our body to greater effect by returning our way of eating to a more natural form.

If you wish to enjoy a long and healthy life free from disease, and to keep your mind sharp and focused throughout, water fasting really is your best bet. It is not a magic pill or a wave of a wand, though, and it will take work and commitment from you. The fact that you have sourced, purchased, and finished reading this book, though, shows an immense drive already. The great sense of achievement that you will experience after your first water fast is phenomenal. As you end each water fast, it is just the beginning of a new season for your body, and as you end this book, your journey begins.

REFERENCES

Alirezaei, M., Kemball, C. C., Flynn, C. T., Wood, M. R., Whitton, J. L., & Kiosses, W. B. (2010, August). Short-term fasting induces profound neuronal autophagy. *Autophagy, 6*(6), 702-710. https://doi.org/10.4161/auto.6.6.12376

Anson, R. M., Guo, Z., de Cabo, R., Iyun, T., Rios, M., Hagepanos, A., ... Mattson, M. P. (2003, May 13). Intermittent fasting dissociates beneficial effects of dietary restriction on glucose metabolism and neuronal resistance to injury from calorie intake. *Proceedings of the National Academy of Sciences of the United States of America, 100*(10), 6216-6220. https://doi.org/10.1073/pnas.1035720100

Beleslin, B., Cirić, J., Zarković, M., Vujović, S., Trbojević, B., & Drezgić, M. (2007). The effects of three-week fasting diet on blood pressure, lipid profile and glucoregulation in extremely obese patients. *Srpski Arhiv Za Celokupno Lekarstvo, 135*(7-8), 440-446. https://doi.org/10.2298/sarh0708440b.

Brandhorst, S., Choi, I. Y., Wei, M., Cheng, C. W., Sedrakyan, S., Navarrete, G., ... Longo, V. D. (2015, July 7). A periodic diet that mimics fasting promotes multi-system regeneration, enhanced cognitive performance, and healthspan. *Cell Metabolism,* 22(1), 86-99. https://doi.org/10.1016/j.cmet.2015.05.012

Gunnars, K. (2019, July 24). *Insulin and insulin resistance - The ultimate guide.* Healthline. https://www.healthline.com/nutrition/insulin-and-insulin-resistance

Hunter, P. (2012, November 6). The inflammation theory of disease. The growing realization that chronic inflammation is crucial in many diseases opens new avenues for treatment. *EMBO Reports, 13*(11), 968-970. https://doi.org/10.1038/embor.2012.142

Kmiec, Z., Pokrywka, L., Kotlarz, G., Kubasik, J., Szutowicz, A., & Mysliwski, A. (2005). Effects of fasting and refeeding on serum leptin, adiponectin and free fatty acid concentrations in young and old male rats. *Gerontology, 51*(6), 357-362. https://doi.org/10.1159/000088698

Lee, J., Duan, W., Long, J. M., Ingram, D. K., & Mattson, M. P. (2000, October). Dietary restriction increases the number of newly generated neural cells, and induces BDNF expression, in the dentate gyrus of rats. *Journal of Molecular*

Neuroscience, 15(2), 99-108. https://doi.org/10.1385/JMN:15:2:99

Levine, B., & Kroemer, G. (2008, January 11). Autophagy in the pathogenesis of disease. *Cell, 132*(1), 27-72. https://doi.org/10.1016/j.cell.2007.12.018

Li, L., Wang, Z., & Zuo, Z. (2013, June 3). Chronic intermittent fasting improves cognitive functions and brain structures in mice. *PloS One, 8*(6), e66069. https://doi.org/10.1371/journal.pone.0066069.

The Nobel Prize in physiology or medicine 2016. (2016). NobelPrize.Org. https://www.nobelprize.org/prizes/medicine/2016/press-release/

Purvis, J. (2009, July 6). Suffragette hunger strikes, 100 years on. *The Guardian*. https://www.theguardian.com/commentisfree/libertycentral/2009/jul/06/suffragette-hunger-strike-protest

Raman, R. (2019, December 18). *Water fasting*. Healthline. https://www.healthline.com/nutrition/water-fasting

Rose, K. (n.d.). *The mental health benefits of fasting*. Amchara. https://www.amchara.com/diet-fasting/the-mental-health-benefits-of-fasting

Salgin, B., (2012, April 1). The effect of prolonged fasting on levels of growth hormone-binding protein and free growth hormone. *Growth Hormone & IGF Research: Official Journal of the Growth Hormone Research Society and the*

International IGF Research Society, 22(2), 76-81. https://doi.org/10.1016/j.ghir.2012.02.003

Short history of fasting. (2017, June 5). Target Health. https://www.targethealth.com/post/short-history-of-fasting

Staff, S. X. (2019, August 22). *Researchers discover that fasting reduces inflammation and improves chronic inflammatory diseases*. Medical Xpress. https://medicalxpress.com/news/2019-08-fasting-inflammation-chronic-inflammatory-diseases.html

Tinsley, G. M., & La Bounty, P. M. (2015, October). Effects of intermittent fasting on body composition and clinical health markers in humans. *Nutrition Reviews, 73*(10), 661-674. https://doi.org/10.1093/nutrit/nuv041

Water fasting (benefits & how to break the fast). (2020, February 4). The LifeCo. https://www.thelifeco.com/en/blog/common-questions-about-water-fasting-benefits-how-to-break-the-fast/

Watson, S. (2020, February 27). *Diabetes: Symptoms, causes, treatment, prevention, and more*. Healthline. https://www.healthline.com/health/diabetes

Wellman, J., (2015). *24 William Secker Quotes*. Christian Quotes. https://www.christianquotes.info/quotes-by-author/william-secker-quotes/

Zauner, C., Schneeweiss, B., Kranz, A., Madl, C., Ratheiser, K., Kramer, L., ... Lenz, K. (2000, June). Resting energy expenditure in short-term starvation is increased as a result of an increase in serum norepinephrine. *The American Journal of Clinical Nutrition, 71*(6), 1511-1515. https://doi.org/10.1093/ajcn/71.6.1511

IMAGE REFERENCE LIST

All images have been sourced from https://pixabay.com

Figure 1: Child Praying. From Pixabay, by Chidioc, 2017. https://pixabay.com/photos/kid-praying-muslim-islam-faith-1077793/

Figure 2: Mineral Water. From Pixabay, by Congerdesign, 2019. https://pixabay.com/photos/bottle-mineral-water-bottle-of-water-2032980/

Figure 3: Pregnancy. From Pixabay, by Free-Photos, 2019. pixabay.com/photos/pregnant-mother-body-pregnant-woman-1245703/

Figure 4: Heart Health. From Pixabay, by InspiredImages, 2017. https://pixabay.com/photos/heart-care-medical-care-heart-1040250/

Figure 5: Yoga. From Pixabay, by StockSnap, 2020. pixabay.-com/photos/people-woman-yoga-meditation-2573216/

Figure 6: Orange Juice. From Pixabay, by Stevepb, 2020. https://pixabay.com/photos/fresh-orange-juice-squeezed-1614822/

Figure 7: Scrambled Eggs. From Pixabay, by Maki_Orel, 2017. https://pixabay.com/photos/breakfast-scrambled-eggs-bun-chive-876432/

Figure 8: Muscle Mass. From Pixabay, by Ryan McGuire, 2019. https://pixabay.com/photos/man-muscle-fitness-workout-641691/

Figure 9: Abdominal Pain. From Pixabay, by Derneuemann, 2020. https://pixabay.com/photos/abdominal-pain-pain-appendicitis-2821941/

Figure 10: Brushing teeth. From Pixabay, by Stevepb, 2020. https://pixabay.com/photos/toothbrush-toothpaste-dental-care-571741/

DOWNLOAD YOUR FREE CHEAT SHEET

(<u>Don't</u> start fasting before you've consulted this cheat sheet...)

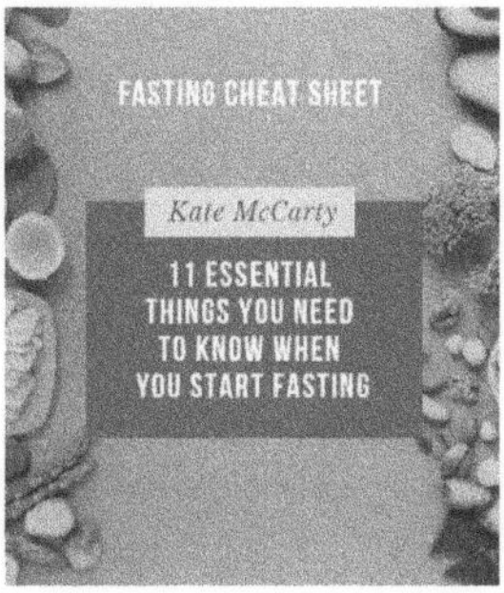

This cheat sheet includes:

- 11 things to know and to do while you are fasting.
- Why you need to know those things to start successfully.
- These things will make the process easier and more enjoyable.

The last thing I want is that the fasting process will be uncomfortable.

To receive your fasting cheat sheet, scan this QR code:

www.ingramcontent.com/pod-product-compliance
Ingram Content Group UK Ltd.
Pitfield, Milton Keynes, MK11 3LW, UK
UKHW041509200225
4680UKWH00031B/607

9 781736 048344